KT-440-426

ILLUSTRATED ELEMENTS OF
TAI CHI

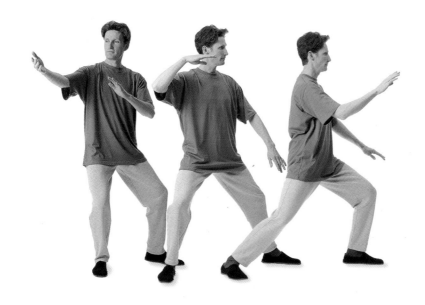

ANGUS CLARK

ELEMENT

First published in 2002 by Element
An imprint of HarperCollins*Publishers*
77–85 Fulham Palace Road
Hammersmith, London W6 8JB

ELEMENT™ is a trademark of HarperCollins*Publishers* Ltd

2 4 6 8 10 9 7 5 3 1

Text copyright © Angus Clark 2002
Copyright © HarperCollins*Publishers* 2002

Angus Clark asserts the moral right to
be identified as the author of this work

This book was created by THE BRIDGEWATER BOOK COMPANY

A catalogue record for this book
is available from the British Library

ISBN 0 00 713386 3

Printed and bound in Hong Kong by Printing Express

All rights reserved. No part of this publication may be
reproduced, stored in a retrieval system, or transmitted,
in any form or by any means, electronic, mechanical,
photocopying, recording or otherwise, without the prior
written permission of the publishers.

NOTE FROM PUBLISHER
Any information given in this book is not intended to be taken
as a replacement for medical advice. Any person with a condition requiring
medical attention should consult a qualified practitioner or therapist.

613 . 7148
CLA

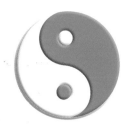

WITHDRAWN

ILLUSTRATED ELEMENTS OF
TAI CHI

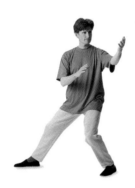

EG29216

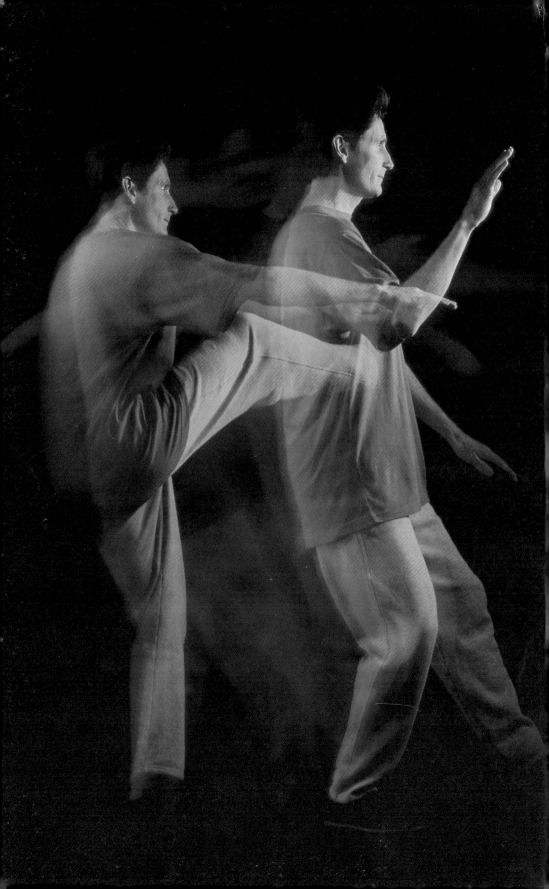

Contents

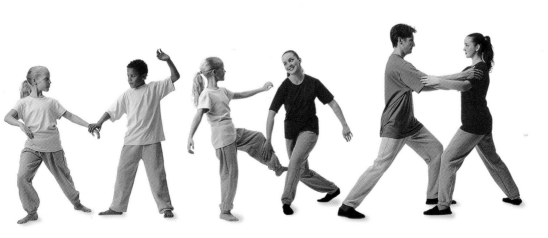

EALING TERTIARY COLLEGE
LEARNING RESOURCE CENTRE - EALING GREEN

Preface

TAI CHI IS *a system of exercises or movements to promote health and longevity, and a comprehensive system of self-defense. Its roots are in China, where it evolved over many hundreds of years as a martial art and as a system of self-development. In the past, many of its techniques were preserved for generations as clan or family secrets, but very gradually, knowledge of the art spread throughout China. Now at the start and end of every day in villages, towns, and cities all over Chinese Asia, people can be seen practicing the slow, graceful movements of tai chi in courtyards, squares, and parks.*

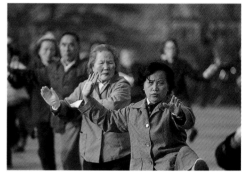

ABOVE *At dawn and as the sun sets in the evening, Chinese people go out to practice tai chi.*

Tai chi was carried to the West in the 20th century, both by Westerners who had studied under Chinese masters, and by Chinese teachers who moved to the West. Nowadays, tai chi is well known in all Western countries, and a wide spectrum of people all over the world practice it regularly. In the West

BELOW *A cascade of cosmic energy sweeps through the body in the Squatting Single Whip posture.*

health organizations, schools, colleges, and even businesses now incorporate tai chi into their curricula and their training programs.

Tai chi is a multidimensional art form that has the capacity to touch several important levels in the life of anyone who embarks on its exploration. Tai chi is not just about health or about self-defense, but about the development of the whole individual – body, mind, and spirit. This book will introduce you to tai chi as a system of movement with a variety of health, fighting, and self-development aspects. The roots of tai chi are ancient, but its principles remain applicable in the highly pressurized modern world.

How to Use this Book

Illustrated Elements of Tai Chi is a comprehensive introduction to an ancient Eastern practice that is becoming more and more popular in the West in response to the pressures of modern life. Tai chi is a holistic healing art that embraces body, mind, and spirit. It improves physical and mental well-being through posture training and exercising all parts of the body, combined with encouraging greater awareness of the links between body and mind. Practiced regularly and with dedication, tai chi becomes a system of self-development and encourages a flowering of personal creativity.

BELOW **The central section of the book takes you step by step through the sequence of movements of the Chen man-ch'ing Short Form.**

BELOW **The book introduces and explains the main body systems, examining the impact of tai chi on the body and the benefits it can bring.**

Thoroughly annotated artworks explain the workings of the body in great detail.

Introductory text explains the role of posture within the Short Form sequence, and examines the benefits it can bring.

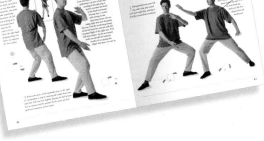

Postures are presented photographically, and flow from page to page in an unbroken sequence.

FOOT DIAGRAMS

Small diagrams explain the foot positions for each posture.

Visualization boxes will give you guidance on your state of mental awareness, helping you to experience the spiritual dimension of tai chi.

RIGHT **The last section of the book explores partner work, the major branches of the art of tai chi, and its role in creativity and self-fulfillment.**

Both feet on the ground

Right heel off the ground

Right foot off the ground

Historical Origins

TAI CHI IS *rooted in the rich soil of ancient Chinese thought, which is based on observing the way things work in nature. The art embodies the concept of continuous change from one extreme to the other as expressed in the ancient book of wisdom, the* I Ching*: "When the sun has reached its meridian, it declines, and when the moon has become full, it wanes." Tai chi stems from the ancient philosophy of Taoism, which arose at a time when China's earliest martial traditions were emerging, among agricultural peoples whose lives were frequently disrupted by wars waged by contending states. And it was founded on the principle of following the natural way or Tao – the ancient philosophy of Taoism.*

ABOVE *The Taoist philosopher Lao Tzu is said to have been Official Archivist of the State of Chou (1st century B.C.E.).*

TAOIST PHILOSOPHY

The first written records of tai chi practice do not appear until the end of the first millennium C.E. However, the art is known to have been developed perhaps a thousand years earlier by Taoist recluses who retreated from the world to mountain hermitages to contemplate the meaning of action by studying nature.

Taoism is an ancient Chinese system of thought that attempts to understand the laws governing change in the universe. The Tao, or Way, is the way the universe works, the natural way of things, from the way the clouds form and disperse to the way a person behaves.

The early Taoists sought to cultivate the Tao within themselves. Taoism centers on the concept of effortless action and the power it engenders. Water symbolizes the idea of strength in weakness; it accepts the lowest level without resistance, yet it wears down the hardest obstacles simply by flowing around them. Striving is the antithe-sis of Taoist action: understanding springs from spontaneous creativity, not from mental or physical effort.

Ideas about the Tao were eventually set down in writing in the *Tao Te Ching* (Classic of the Way and Virtue), the principal text of Taoism, an anthology of writings produced in about 300 B.C.E. (often referred to as the *Lao Tzu*).

The philosophers of ancient China sought to make suggestions that might generate ideas and unanswered questions in the mind. Taoist writings are full of paradoxes and contradictions intended to challenge limited and inhibiting views on life, and to open the perceptions.

Taoist thought pervades tai chi. "Plants when they enter life are soft and tender," says the *Lao Tzu*. "When they die they are dry and stiff... The hard and strong are companions of death. The soft and weak are the companions of life." In tai chi, learning the qualities of softness and understanding its power are essential parts of practice.

TAI AND CHI

In Chinese, the characters for "tai" and "chi" express a double superlative, often translated as "Supreme Ultimate" or more simply as "cosmos." Tai chi is said to have been born from *wu chi*, the Great Void, the original state of cosmic emptiness. With the birth of tai chi, stillness changed into movement or energy. This movement was generated by the interplay of the opposing yet complementary forces of yin and yang (opposite). Tai chi can also be interpreted as "central pole" or "pillar," like the ridgepole of a house around which all the other parts are arranged and upon which they all depend. T'ai chi is a Western abbreviation of the Chinese term *tai chi ch'uan*, the full name of the Chinese fighting art. which translated means "fighting art based on the laws of the universe."

CHANGE AND HARMONY

Chinese philosophy is based on a belief in two opposing but complementary forces, yin and yang. Traditionally, yin has been presented as the feminine force, passive, nurturing, and soft, and yang as the harder, more active masculine principle. Yin and yang are also the forces of harmony and change, and together they form a balanced whole. When they are not in perfect equilibrium, disorder and disease are said to follow. The interrelationship between change and harmony is the guiding principle behind tai chi, which seeks to establish a dynamic equilibrium between the two.

Change is a constant in our lives. The Earth moves unceasingly around its orbit, causing the seasons to change and recreating the cycle of birth, life, and death. From the moment of conception to the time of death the body changes ceaselessly. The blood circulates, air is breathed in and out, mind and body mature and age. Throughout our lives we experience not one moment of absolute stillness. Change brings about rhythm, however – every in-breath is followed by an out-breath – and so harmony is maintained.

This ceaseless interplay between change and harmony is perfectly expressed in the yin-yang symbol (above). As any condition reaches its fullest point, it already contains the seed of its opposite: in the dark portion is a seed of white; and in the white portion is a seed of black.

In tai chi the interplay between yin and yang, the forces of change and harmony, reveals itself in the changing postures and the quality of the movements. Body weight shifts from one leg to the other, awareness moves from inside to out, empty changes to full, open to closed. The forces work simultaneously, creating a continous and ever-changing dance of energy. Life is filled with countless forces and arrangements of opposites: day and night; sound and silence; giving and receiving; fear and courage; sadness and happiness. Taoism teaches that the concepts of yin and yang offer a view of the way things work according to a natural law of change and harmony.

Everyone practicing tai chi is enjoined to embody natural law in their movements in accordance with the constantly changing balance between yin and yang. It may take time, practice, concentration, and self-love, but the reward is true harmony of body and mind, the achievement of central equilibrium – which is the essence of tai chi.

YIN YANG QUALITIES

Below is a list of a few of the many yin and yang qualities. It is important, however, not to see any of them as always being a yin or a yang quality, but as generally belonging to either category under certain circumstances. For example, the Earth receives the seed, protects it, and nurtures it, and so is usually categorized as yin, but if you fall and hit the ground you experience it as hard – as yang.

Yin	Yang
Inward	Outward
Smooth	Rough
Holding	Sending
Receiving	Giving
Listening	Speaking
Dark	Light
Earth	Sky
Soft	Hard
No boundaries	Clear boundaries

THE I CHING

The *I Ching* or *Book of Changes* is the classic of Taoist thought. It is a book of divination and wisdom, stemming from oracles written more than 4,000 years ago. The *I Ching* is a collection of commentaries on 64 hexagrams. Hexagrams are drawn by tossing coins. You ask the book a question on any subject, and its answer appears in the hexagram you drew. The text interprets life conditions and situations in terms of yin and yang. Many people find the *I Ching* assists in their decisions by helping them to make wise choices.

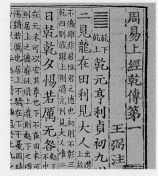

ABOVE *The hexagram Chien from a copy of the* I Ching *printed in China in the tenth century* B.C.E.

The Birth of Tai Chi

ONE TRADITION SAYS *that tai chi originated some 5,000 years ago during the reign of China's mythical first emperor, Fu Hsi. Exercises for health are described in a collection of classic writings attributed to one of his successors, the legendary Yellow Emperor, Huang Ti, who is said to have founded the traditional Chinese system of medicine. The principles of the art were established by Taoist recluses who retired from the world to live as hermits. And it evolved during turbulent periods in China's history as a martial art called t'ai chi ch'uan.*

Although tai chi is thought to have originated before the first millennium, the earliest known references date from the T'ang Dynasty (618–960 C.E.). They describe "patterns" of tai chi practiced by recluses who had retired to China's mountain regions.

The early tai chi teachers remain semi-mythical figures. Chang San-feng is no exception, a colorful figure, said to have been more than 6

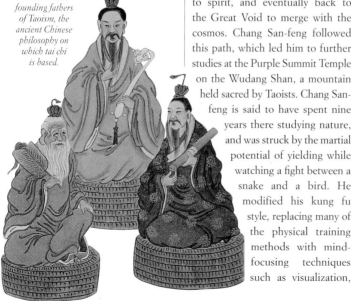

RIGHT *Three founding fathers of Taoism, the ancient Chinese philosophy on which tai chi is based.*

feet tall and a powerful fighter. No one knows whether he really existed or when he lived. Yet, he is credited as the founder of a spiritual fighting art called Wudang kung fu.

History records that Chang San-feng studied under a Taoist recluse living in the northwest of China, then studied martial arts at the Shaolin Temple Monastery near Zhengzhou in modern Henan.

It is said that in tai chi a process leads the player from body to mind to spirit, and eventually back to the Great Void to merge with the cosmos. Chang San-feng followed this path, which led him to further studies at the Purple Summit Temple on the Wudang Shan, a mountain held sacred by Taoists. Chang San-feng is said to have spent nine years there studying nature, and was struck by the martial potential of yielding while watching a fight between a snake and a bird. He modified his kung fu style, replacing many of the physical training methods with mind-focusing techniques such as visualization,

and the cultivation of energy through qigung. From this point, China's "soft" fighting arts – ba gua, hsingi, and t'ai chi ch'uan – developed.

As the peaceful and prosperous Ming Dynasty declined in the 1600s, to be replaced by conquerors from Manchuria, hand-to-hand battlefield combat was a frequent reality and personal combat skills were at a premium. Foremost among the soft, or internal, fighting styles was the Chen style of tai chi, founded by Chen Wang-t'ing, a soldier in the imperial Ming armies who served under a respected general, Ch'i Chi-guang. Ch'i wrote the *Classic of kung fu,* setting out the principles of what became Chen style. However, it is also claimed that Chen studied under the author of the now-classic *Treatise on T'ai Chi Ch'uan,* Wang Tsung-yueh, whose lineage could be traced back to the legendary fighter Chang San-feng.

By the 1800s tai chi was at its zenith as a fighting art, and the Chen style was well established. However, it was still taught only to members of the Chen family. In the early 1800s a student from a poor family, Yang Lu-ch'an, worked in the household of the clan head, Chen Chang-xing. where he spied on tai chi sessions. One day he offered to fight a stranger who had challenged Chen Chang-xing. Yang fought so well that it was obvious that he had been secretly learning the Chen style. Chen accepted Yang as a student.

Yang Lu-ch'an traveled China as a Chen family representative, offering challenges to fighters, and was nicknamed "Ever-Victorious." He is said to have been appointed to teach Chen-style t'ai chi ch'uan to the household of the Ch'ing Emperor. Chen style is dynamic and physically demanding. To adapt the style for courtiers who had not trained from early youth Yang omitted the more vigorous movements, creating a gentler form of tai chi. Today, while Chen is recognized as the oldest of the three main tai chi styles practiced today, a shorter version of Yang's style is most widely taught.

An outstanding teacher who bridged the classic tai chi styles with 20th century development is Cheng Man-ching. In the 1930's Cheng, a disciple of Yang Cheng Fu, condensed his teacher's form of 108 moves down to a more managable 37. He opened a school in New York in the 1960's and as a result was most instrumental in bringing tai chi to West. Another short version of the Yang style was created in 1949 by the Washu Council of China, known as the Peking 24 step.

The third style was developed by Yang's student, Wu Yu-hsiang, who also studied with the Chen family, so his style incorporates features of both. These three styles have given rise to numerous derivatives.

TAI CHI SPREADS WORLDWIDE

During the 1800s t'ai chi ch'uan flourished and the classic schools were established. New warfare technology diminished tai chi's role as a battlefield art so that the tai chi families no longer needed to keep their arts secret. Since 1900 tai chi has become accessible to ordinary Chinese people, and has spread westward, to North America, Australia and New Zealand, and into Europe.

Early 1800s
Yang Lu-ch'an becomes the first non-family member to study Chen Old Form under Chen Chang-hsing.

1880s
Chinese emigrants carry tai chi and other martial arts to Southeast Asia.

SINGAPORE

Mid 1800s
Yang Lu-ch'an founds the Yang style.

Wu Yu-hsiang founds the first Wu style.

Late 1800s
Li Yi-yu and Hou Wei-chen modify Old Wu style to found the Li or Hou Style.

Tientsin 1900
The Boxer Uprising, an anti-foreign rebellion, is put down by Western troops with guns.

1949
China's Communist government establishes the Peking 24, 36, 48, and 88 step forms.

1920s
Yang Cheng-fu, grandson of Yang Lu-ch'an, develops Yang-style Big Form, marking the start of recreational tai chi.

Sun Lu-t'ang, a master of Chinese martial arts, founds Sun Style.

PEKING (BEIJING)

TIANJIN

KOREA

HENAN

EAST CHINA SEA

1930s
Cheng Man-ch'ing transforms the classic Yang Big Style into the 37-step Short Form.

CHEKIANG PROVINCE

TAIPEI

TAIWAN

1970s
Dr. Chi Chiang-tao teaches his variation on Cheng Man-ch'ing's Short Form in the UK.

1968–72
Cheng Man-ch'ing founds a tai chi school in New York.

Mid-1900s
Cheng Man-ch'ing leaves China and founds a tai chi school in Taipei.

CAMBRIDGE

NEW YORK

SAN FRANCISCO

LONDON

CHINA IN THE 1800S   EXTENT OF BOXER UPRISING

A Healing Art

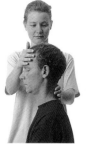

TAI CHI IS *best known in the West as a system of exercises to benefit health, prevent degenerative illnesses, and promote longevity. It stimulates circulation, aligns misplaced bones, mobilizes the joints, stimulates and maintains vital organs, and improves balance and coordination. It improves the breathing, which revitalizes body and brain. But tai chi is a holistic practice and it also trains the mind to focus and concentrate. It widens sensitivity and the capacity to feel, so that people who practice become more awake, alive, and responsive.*

ABOVE *A few minutes of gentle massage can release tension and remove pain.*

The following pages show many different ways in which tai chi can benefit health of body and mind. Tai chi works with the body to support and encourage its natural capacity for healing. Practicing the techniques correctly raises chi, or life energy, which strengthens the immune system and improves health, and jin or whole body energy, also called intrinsic energy, which improves coordination.

Tai chi movements build energy gradually. Tai chi movements generate warmth, often accompanied by a sense of fullness. After perhaps half an hour of practice the body may feel as if it is humming. After a training session this can be felt as heat energy in certain parts of the body, especially the hands, which seem to radiate heat.

When tai chi is practiced regularly, a combination of mindset, visualization, body shape (the positions made by the body), and movement create the conditions for streams of energy to flow vigorously through the body, stimulating the internal systems. It is said in the ancient writings on tai chi that the chi (life energy) follows the mind – each posture cultivates a different kind of energy flow, depending on visualization and the body shapes it makes. The hands are transmitters for this energy, and become charged by the large amounts of information that pass through them.

Healing is a natural force that cannot be made to take place, any more than a plant can be made to grow. The role of the individual in the process is to try, through tai chi, to create the conditions in which energy can flow, and to give the body time to heal itself.

HEALING OTHERS

Massage for tai chi can be reassuring, so offering to massage relatives or friends is a way of helping them through touch. Explore the following methods for yourself and discover how the healing energy generated in tai chi practice can help you, your friends, and family.

Foot-holding and intuitive foot massage

The simple technique of foot-holding embodies the principle of "not doing" perfectly. For the best effect the person to be massaged should lie down comfortably, or, if this is not possible, sit in a chair with the knees and legs supported on a stool or cushions. Rest your hands on the other person's ankles or feet and do nothing for at least 10 minutes. Notice how energy builds in both bodies.

This demonstrates the two-way nature of healing and the positive feedback that begins with tai chi practice. Intuitive foot massage is stimulating and comforting. Simply massage the other person's feet in any way that occurs to you.

Dispelling a headache

Ask your friend to sit comfortably. Rest your right hand on his or her forehead and your left hand on the back of the neck, and keep your hands still for at least three minutes. Now move your hands about 9 inches away from your friend's head and neck, imagining them offering a healing space into which the "disease" of the headache can melt. Finish by placing both of your hands in light contact with your friend's head for about a minute.

MASSAGE

The idea in massage for tai chi is to develop your spontaneity and intuition for self-healing. There are no special strokes to apply, and you need not worry about direction or pressure of stroke. Begin by following your own feelings about what to do. Rub briskly if you want to, or stroke gently.

MASSAGING THE FACE
Bring both hands to your chin and slowly draw them up over your face, back through your hair, and down your neck. Repeat five times.

MASSAGING THE EARS
Rub the lobes of each ear vigorously, then run your finger and thumb around the rim of the ear and back again to each ear lobe.

MASSAGING THE EYES
Close your eyes and (always with clean hands) stroke the upper eyelids lightly with the middle finger from close to the top of the nose out to the side of the head. Repeat this action at least seven times, then stroke the bottom eyelid in the same way.

MASSAGING THE FEET
Massaging your feet stimulates the nerve-endings and is relaxing and comforting. Hold or rub your feet one at a time for at least two minutes each.

RIGHT The feet work hard, yet they tend to be neglected. They benefit from massage, especially before and after practice.

MASSAGING THE HANDS
Massage stimulates the many nerve-endings in the hands, improving the circulation and bringing life to them. Gently or vigorously rub your hands. Pay attention to each finger and both thumbs, the palms, and the backs of the hands.

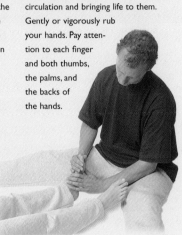

SELF-HEALING

Tai chi is a healing art and just practicing it generates the energy that makes healing possible. The following exercises act as a useful complement to this aspect of tai chi. They can be done at any time, but they are especially effective immediately after practice.

HANDS ON
1 Place your left hand on the lower tantien energy center, just below the navel, and your right hand on top of it. Rest in this position for two to five minutes. Concentrate on gathering into yourself and recharging your batteries.

HANDS ON
2 Release your hands, place your right hand on the lower tantien and your left hand on the center of your chest. Again, hold this position for two to five minutes, concentrating on gathering into yourself and charging your batteries.

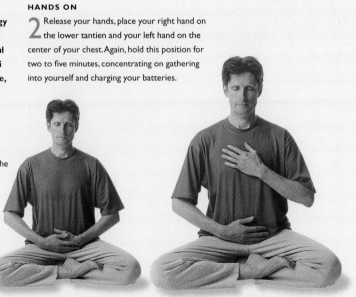

Seven Qualities

EVERY POSTURE IN *tai chi is a combination of seven basic qualities. Central to these qualities is the concept of yin and yang, the forces of change and harmony. Like yin and yang, the basic qualities of tai chi are almost all polarities: open and closed; full and empty. The exception is the seventh, central equilibrium. Consciousness of these seven qualities pervades every aspect of a posture. They are the focus of the mind, they are expressed in the movements, and they are the message communicated through the very spirit of the posture.*

The nonstop sequence of movements called the form is the essence of the art of tai chi. The postures are in a state of perpetual transformation, a cycle of harmony and change. A posture begins, grows, reaches a fullness, and starts to empty, ready for the growth of the next one.

To fulfil their task of restoring equilibrium between yin and yang, the movements of the form must be executed with the correct technique and mind intent (attitude). Often for a beginner, body and mind are too fully occupied with learning the sequence of movements and the technique to experience the qualities of each movement. So, to accompany the form practice, experiment with moves that develop a sense of feeling, such as relaxing your muscles and moving your weight from one side to the other.

All postures contain the polarities of open and closed. Open is

generally associated with gathering energy and closed with releasing. At each moment every part of the body is either open or closed, so studying one's own posture helps in understanding the concept. Bringing the hands together as if clapping, carries the feeling of closed. Open is felt

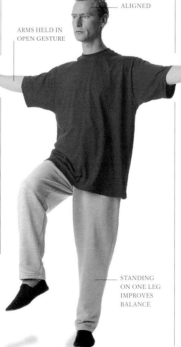

BODY ALIGNED

ARMS HELD IN OPEN GESTURE

STANDING ON ONE LEG IMPROVES BALANCE

RIGHT *Balance improves by standing on each leg in turn for a few minutes each day. This strengthens the legs and improves the coordination, but it also makes you feel different. Physical equilibrium infiltrates the mental and emotional spheres of your being.*

when lifting the arms outward as when welcoming friends.

The polarities of full and empty give the body mobility. In tai chi balance is held in one side, leaving the other free to move. The balance empties from one side and fills the other, as the exercise Balanced Walking (page 54) demonstrates, increasing mobility. Open or closed, the body must be in balance.

Without equilibrium a posture will lose its structure, becoming too open or too closed. Structure lends strength to a posture. Central equilibrium is the foundation of every stance and the hub of every movement. When a posture is based on central equilibrium, the body is aligned between earth and sky, so it is perfectly balanced.

Beginners unfamiliar with these ideas find it hard to combine the mental concept with the physical experience. Familiarity makes these qualities more and more interesting, however, since they affect almost every aspect of every tai chi movement. Familiarizing yourself with them therefore needs to become part of regular practice.

EXPERIENCE YOUR BODY SHAPES

Create your own body shapes to express the qualities of yin and yang described on page 9. As a guide for yin, use soft, round, smooth, flowing shapes to embody the qualities. For yang use hard, angular, and linear shapes as your guiding concepts. Play with all these possibilities and add your own movements.

You can discover how open and closed feel when expressed as movement. As you practice, the polarity intensifies the experience of the movement.

The second exercise expands the first to make greater demands on your imagination. Imagine yourself as an empty vessel; picture the reality of fullness.

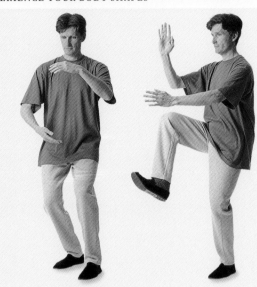

YIN BODY SHAPE   YANG BODY SHAPE

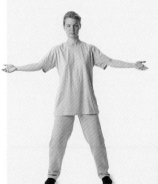
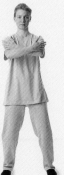
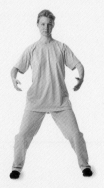
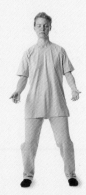

OPEN AND CLOSED

1 Stand with your feet apart, lift your arms up and out in a welcoming gesture, and imagine each body part and your feelings opening up.

OPEN AND CLOSED

2 Slowly draw your arms in, crossing them over your chest, contemplating this closed position. End by lowering your arms and standing erect for a while.

FULL AND EMPTY

1 Imagine colored liquid filling you from your feet up. Experience every cell in your body expanding as it rises, moving your arms out as if you are inflating.

FULL AND EMPTY

2 Then close your eyes and imagine your body is hollow. Visualize yourself becoming emptiness.

Seven Steps to Progress

TAI CHI OFFERS *more than exercises for health, it also provides a program for self-development. The influential teachers Cheng Man-ch'ing and Chi Chiang-tao mapped out a sevenfold path to tai chi practice. For just as the postures are composed of seven basic qualities, so there are seven dimensions to practice, seven steps to progress through the form.*

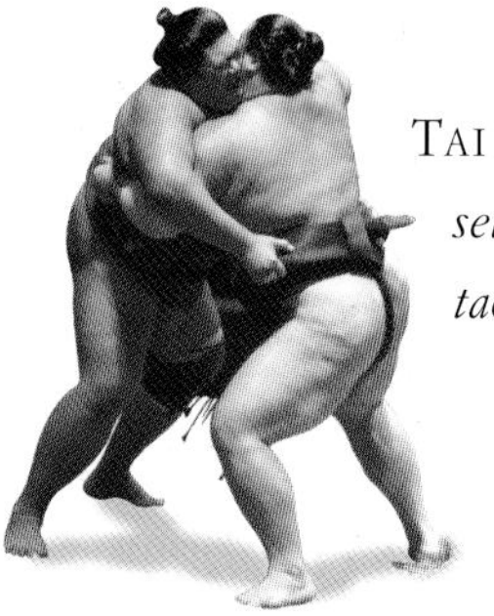

LEFT *Tai chi teaches you to respond to a partner's movements. Sumo wrestlers use force against force.*

Imagine trying to stop the flow of a river or make it flow faster. The way of tai chi is always to flow with the river. Beginners may be surprised to find that they have been conditioned to fight the river's natural flow, to use force against force. We are trained to keep to timetables and meet deadlines rather than follow the natural rhythms of our body and mind.

Tai chi teaches people to correct this imbalance by becoming alert to intelligence from within while learning to listen to what is happening outside and to respond to others. It

MAPPING TAI CHI PRACTICE

The seven dimensions of tai chi practice, described on the page opposite, may be represented by a graph on which you map your progress along the path to natural way. The vertical axis measures your progress on a scale from 1 to 10. A teacher might help you assess your abilities in each area. Draw a new graph to review progress after a year. Your tendency to use force against force should have fallen and your energy and coordination have risen.

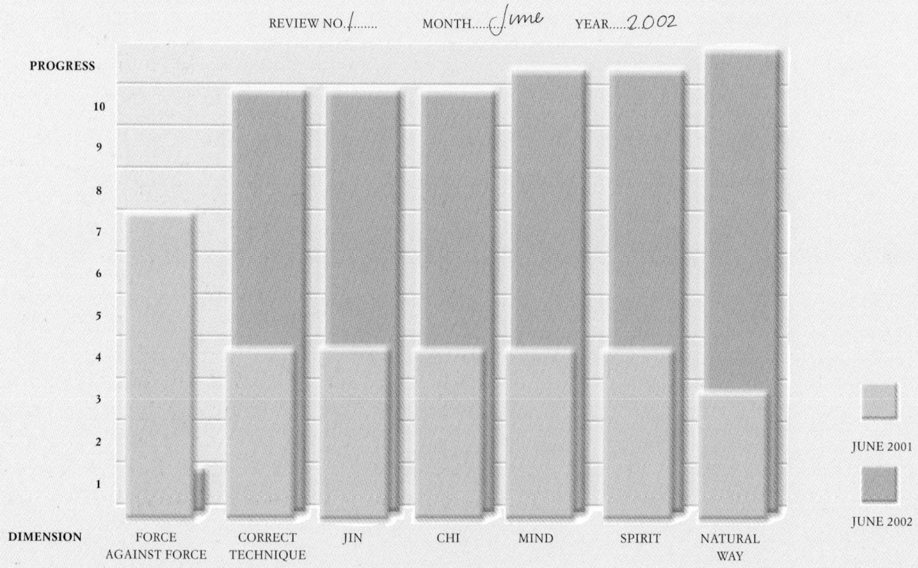

REVIEW NO. *1*   MONTH *June*   YEAR *2002*

PROGRESS

DIMENSION: FORCE AGAINST FORCE · CORRECT TECHNIQUE · JIN · CHI · MIND · SPIRIT · NATURAL WAY

JUNE 2001

JUNE 2002

teaches patience, the ability to wait, poised and quiet, for the right moment to move or act.

When tai chi movements are performed correctly, they work to calm and focus the mind, so that mind, energy, and body work in harmony. The seven dimensions of tai chi practice are described below, and represented on the graph (left).

FORCE AGAINST FORCE

Are you trying to dominate by blocking your partner's responses, or responding too quickly, before your partner stops pushing? If so, you are using force against force. In this interaction you enter into a dialog, inviting your partner to respond to your push. Do not try to force one. When receiving a push, listen as the movement unfolds, knowing that each push has its lifetime. Do not stop it by force, but move in response to the other person. This is the natural way.

CORRECT TECHNIQUE

Although the rules of tai chi are challenging, they are effective. Hands and feet need to be correctly aligned, placed, and arranged; doing this enables you to reap the richest reward from practice. And bear in mind that improvement often comes without a struggle. Working on the mind, for instance, sharpens concentration, which brings about improvements in technique.

JIN OR WHOLE BODY ENERGY

Beginners feel all left feet. As practice evolves, feet, legs and pelvis, spine, arms, and hands feel more con-

nected, and movements of head and body begin to feel coordinated. There comes a time when breathing and movement of all parts of the body follow one rhythm, and this cohesion is jin (whole body energy).

CHI OR LIFE FORCE ENERGY

Tai chi movements stimulate the chi circulating in the body and the musculoskeletal system, exercise the internal organs, and open the meridians (see page 40), allowing chi to build. Resting the mind quietly in the lower tantien energy center (see page 45) after practice also builds chi. People often feel contentment and greater vitality after practice.

MIND

Cultivating awareness is the key to mind control – if your mind keeps returning to one of the day's events while you are practicing, acknowledge it. Notice where your mind is directed as you move. Soon, there will be moments when it becomes absorbed in the moves you are making, and the moments will extend to minutes. Then you find your mind making visualizations at will.

SPIRIT

There is a dynamic equilibrium between earth and spirit in tai chi. The way to spirit is through the earthing of the body, and the stronger the connection with the earth, the greater the possibilities for spirit. One of the joys of practice is allowing the body to radiate the spirit that powers each posture – the spirit of fire or of clarity. Enjoy the spirit of the moment; you may feel

MIND GAME

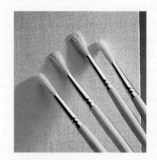

This visualization may take a while to become real, but it will show how your mind and your energy can work together. Turn your left palm toward you. Point the fingers of your right hand toward your left palm keeping them about six inches away. Imagine the fingers of your right hand are brushes. Paint strokes very slowly over your left hand. At first you may not sense anything, but soon you will feel the light brush strokes moving across the sensitive palm of your hand as clearly as if you were really painting it.

poised, like a cat about to pounce, then you might become quiet, nurturing the spirit inside.

NATURAL WAY

Follow the natural way to emerge into the seventh dimension. Let go of the binding patterns of force against force, become receptive to the natural way of things, and learn to wait for the right moment to move. Attaining natural way is a sevenfold process. The qualities work together to realign the whole person toward natural way.

Movement, Health, and Body Awareness

THE BODY IS *an extraordinary, wonderful instrument. It is mechanically well designed and physically intricate, yet it also houses the spirit. The body bestows on its owner the gift of movement, yet people living a modern lifestyle rarely if ever make the most of this ability, and many have forgotten or never discovered their bodies' capabilities. Yet not only is the body designed to move, it needs to, in order to stay healthy. Tai chi provides a form of exercise that offers a remedy for the ills of modern living, a supportive answer to the body's need to move.*

While they are still developing in their mother's womb, unborn infants know how to move. They swim, dance, push, wriggle, and kick. Immediately after birth, babies move instinctively and without inhibition, and during the early years, movement plays an essential part in childhood learning and personal development. Young children crawl, roll, totter, and fall; as they grow they play on swings, slides, roundabouts, and with each other. A child's world is largely body-based.

Relatively few adults in modern industrial countries still have to cut hay, harvest crops, fetch water, or chop wood by hand in order to survive. Most are relieved of such tiresome tasks and chores by modern economic organization, which uses machines to perform repetitive jobs, releasing people to attend to tasks carried out by telephone, pager, fax, or computer, reached by automobile, rail or air link, e-mail or internet. Many are not forced by their work to stretch or stress their bodies. Problems tend to begin shortly after the point where demands cease to be

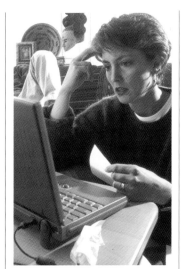

ABOVE *A sedentary lifestyle now can mean mobility problems later on in life.*

made of the body. Arthritis, for example, is associated with under-exercising the joints. One physiologist has estimated that 150 years of good service could normally be expected from the superbly designed joints of the human frame. Yet they waste away, working at a fraction of their potential, while the body sits on office chairs or lounges on sofas.

By placing emphasis on mental achievement and a globalizing electronic culture, contemporary living draws energy from the body into the head, simply because exercising the mind draws blood to the brain. The ratio of mental and emotional stimulation to physical activity was reversed during the 20th century, and for many the reversal took place in fewer than 50 years. Modern work stresses the mind but fails to work the body, making true rest difficult to achieve.

Western society today is predominantly sedentary. Anyone doing an office or a driving job is required to sit for long periods. Then, at the end of the day they rest in a sitting position, unlike most animals, which tend to rest lying down. Tribal peoples who retain their ancient customs often rest by squatting, kneeling, or lying. Modern people sit on a chair, on the tail of the spine, a position that far from being restful is a kind of slump. In time, this bad posture can result in a tendency to asthma, lower back trouble, and prolapsed (displaced) internal organs.

Sitting back to relax and watch TV sets up another dynamic. The body responds to the visual stimuli presented on a screen by producing an emotional response in the form of energy that needs to find expression. Aware of the need for an outlet for such unexpressed energy, many people take up some form of exercise. It is all too easy, however, to overreact and pummel the body with exercise. Activity that is too vigorous can shock the body and injure its systems.

HEAD AND SPINE ALIGNED

OPEN ARMS

ABOVE *Tai chi is a holistic practice, its movements exercise the whole body, not just individual muscles or muscle groups. It works gently to encourage the body's natural harmony.*

BALANCED STANCE

Tai chi is quality movement. It is physically demanding, yet it works with the body to encourage the gradual developing of strength and reviving of natural openness and coordination. This process is not something that can be hurried, however. Tai chi is an art that needs to be mastered through gradual learning and practice, but the benefits of investing time and effort in it become apparent very early on.

Like a door, the body must be kept moving to prevent its hinge joints – and other types of joint – from seizing up, and tai chi works to condition the elements of the human frame. It promotes greater understanding of the body's natural alignment and stance, encouraging the habit of good posture. Its movements continually turn the spine, an action that gradually repositions misplaced organs, stimulating them at the same time through an internal form of massage. The tai chi movements dissipate excess nervous tension held in the body and so help balance the nervous system. Through apparently simple exercises, such as standing on one leg, tai chi stimulates the muscle groups to work together. Continued through life it prevents the joints of the hips and limbs from degenerating.

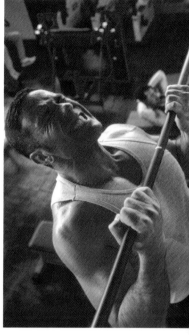

ABOVE *Working out can demand too much of the body without considering its needs and tolerances.*

The unique upright stance of humans gives us a greater potential for movements than creatures who walk on four legs. The physical capabilities of humans may seem inferior when in water, yet it is the human who can walk out of the water onto the land, play volleyball, climb a tree, paint a picture, and cook a meal. Each day, our bodies perform wonders for us.

But do we know our bodies? The next few pages present some of the workings of the body from a holistic point of view, from the mechanical structure of the frame to the internal systems and the location of the energy centers, and show how tai chi encourages the development of a personal connection with the body.

The Skeleton

THE BODY'S ARCHITECTURE *provides the framework for the extraordinary variety of movement and bodily expression that is tai chi. The art makes full use of the combination of dexterity, flexibility, articulation, and movement capabilities that the skeleton, aided by ligaments, muscles, and tendons, makes possible. Knowing the basics of body architecture will deepen understanding of the tai chi postures. It will also give a sense of wonder at the sheer variety of movements the human body can perform, unparalleled in the rest of the animal kingdom.*

The skeleton is the body's frame, supporting it and giving it shape. The bony cavities of the skull, the rib cage, and the pelvic girdle provide protection for the body's vital organs – the brain, the lungs, the organs of digestion, and the sexual organs. Design of the skeleton has evolved over millions of years to make it perfectly adapted for movement. The girders of a building are bolted into a rigid framework, but the skeletal bones are connected by joints held together by ligaments and operated by muscles. This system gives the body mobility.

Tai chi actively increases mobility in all the joints of the body, maintaining an especially strong focus on the ankles, knees, hips, shoulders, elbows, wrists, and spine. It achieves this mainly by encouraging the joints to open, that is, to relax completely (see page 15).

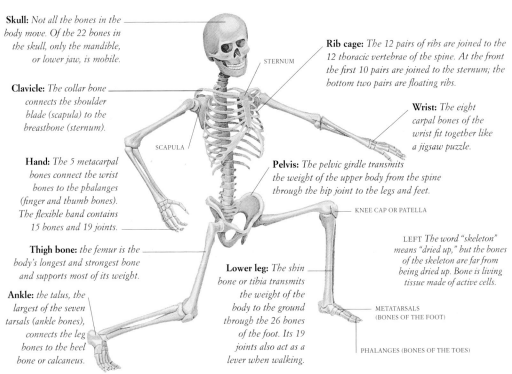

Skull: *Not all the bones in the body move. Of the 22 bones in the skull, only the mandible, or lower jaw, is mobile.*

Clavicle: *The collar bone connects the shoulder blade (scapula) to the breastbone (sternum).*

Hand: *The 5 metacarpal bones connect the wrist bones to the phalanges (finger and thumb bones). The flexible hand contains 15 bones and 19 joints.*

Thigh bone: *the femur is the body's longest and strongest bone and supports most of its weight.*

Ankle: *the talus, the largest of the seven tarsals (ankle bones), connects the leg bones to the heel bone or calcaneus.*

STERNUM

SCAPULA

Lower leg: *The shin bone or tibia transmits the weight of the body to the ground through the 26 bones of the foot. Its 19 joints also act as a lever when walking.*

Rib cage: *The 12 pairs of ribs are joined to the 12 thoracic vertebrae of the spine. At the front the first 10 pairs are joined to the sternum; the bottom two pairs are floating ribs.*

Wrist: *The eight carpal bones of the wrist fit together like a jigsaw puzzle.*

Pelvis: *The pelvic girdle transmits the weight of the upper body from the spine through the hip joint to the legs and feet.*

KNEE CAP OR PATELLA

LEFT *The word "skeleton" means "dried up," but the bones of the skeleton are far from being dried up. Bone is living tissue made of active cells.*

METATARSALS (BONES OF THE FOOT)

PHALANGES (BONES OF THE TOES)

Bone is living tissue made of active cells served by blood vessels and nerves, and the tissues in its spongy center carry out the vital task of making bone marrow. The red blood cells, which transport oxygen, are formed in the bone marrow along with white blood cells, which fight infection. Bones are fundamental to the body's immune system.

Tai chi attributes another important function to the bone marrow. The teacher Cheng Man-ch'ing described the cultivation of chi in the lower tantien energy center, how it warms the fluids of the body and fills the hollow spaces of the bones. An adhesive substance forms, which turns into marrow and plates the insides of the bones like nickel or gold, giving them greater weight and pure hardness.

THE BONES

All bones begin as flexible cartilage, which forms in the womb. As the baby grows the cartilage is gradually converted into bones, which continue to lengthen and grow until the end of the teen years. A baby's skeleton has more than 350 bones, many of which eventually fuse, so that an adult's skeleton has only 206 bones.

THE SPINE

The spine is made up of 33 bones but only 25 joints because the last four bones are fused to form the coccyx (tail bone) and the five bones above them are fused to form the sacrum. Each bone is called a vertebra, and the vertebrae form groups, each of which differs slightly in its function. The vertebrae are separated by disks of cartilage, forming a

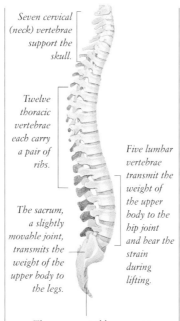

Seven cervical (neck) vertebrae support the skull.

Twelve thoracic vertebrae each carry a pair of ribs.

The sacrum, a slightly movable joint, transmits the weight of the upper body to the legs.

Five lumbar vertebrae transmit the weight of the upper body to the hip joint and bear the strain during lifting.

The coccyx or tail bone consists of five fused bones. Like the sacrum, it moves only during pregnancy.

ABOVE *The bones, or vertebrae, and joints of the spine.*

slightly movable joint. These cartilaginous joints work together, allowing the spine to move forward, backward, and sideways. The spinal cord, a bundle of major nerve fibers, travels along a channel through the center of the vertebrae from the pelvis to join the brain.

THE SACRUM

The broad shield-shaped bone at the base of the spine transmits the weight of the body from the fifth lumbar vertebra sideways to the pelvic girdle. The sacrum "sacred bone" forms the bottom bend of the spine's s-curve. It forms a slightly movable joint with the fifth lumbar

vertebra, but its side "wings" fit perfectly into the corresponding surfaces of the pelvic girdle, and ligaments secure the sacroiliac joints so firmly they are almost immobile. The sacrum is fundamental to the mechanics of tai chi movement.

THE JOINTS

The body has many other moving joints (see below). Although tai chi movements exercise all the body's joints, they focus on opening and exercising the joints of the ankles, knees, hips, shoulders, elbows, and wrists, and on maintaining the mobility of the multi-jointed spine.

Ball and socket joint
A ball and socket joint is where the rounded head of one bone fits into a socket or hole in the adjoining bone. Ball and socket joints at the shoulders and hip allow the arms and legs almost 360° of movement.

Hinge joint
The knee, toes, fingers, and elbow are examples of hinge joints, which permit bending and straightening in one direction. A rounded bulge in one bone fits into a corresponding hollow in an adjoining bone. The two bones are held together by ligaments and encased in a capsule filled with a lubricating fluid.

Pivot joint
The first two cervical vertebrae in the neck form a pivot joint. A protuberance in the second cervical vertebra, called the axis, fits into a ring formed in the vertebra above it, called the atlas, allowing the neck to pivot from side to side.

The Muscles

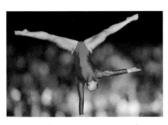

ABOVE *Gymnasts may seem to achieve the impossible, but they are in fact demonstrating the full flexibility that the skeletal muscles can achieve.*

ONE OF THE *first things people notice when they start tai chi is that their legs begin to feel different. To some it can be a shock to find that the gentle, flowing movements, so attractive to watch, can require such hard work from the muscles of their thighs and calves. But it is the demands made on the muscle groups of the legs combined with the ability to fully relax muscles elsewhere in the body that gives tai chi its unique grace of movement.*

We often need to retrain some of the muscles under our conscious control through tai chi, especially those of the lower limbs, which play a major role in bodily expression. For this reason, after a tai chi posture is learned there may be a time-gap before it can be performed with real ease. This is the maturing time the muscles need to strengthen and learn the new movements.

The muscles execute commands from the brain carried along the motor nerves. For the muscles to be able to react so quickly, the nervous system maintains them in a half-alert state called muscle tone, ensuring that voluntary movements are not started from cold.

This link with the nervous system means that emotional stress registers in the muscles, however. Feelings of fear or anxiety show as a measurable rise in muscle tone. This reaction is appropriate as a "fight-or-flight" response, enabling the body to react instantly to an emergency, but people who suffer from recurrent fear or anxiety may be held in a per-

manent state of tension and find it hard to rest and impossible to relax, a state of chronic stress,

On one level tai chi deals with stress by relaxing the muscles. "Soft" does not mean flaccid, but a way of using muscles exactly as required for each movement. This allows a release of unnecessary muscular tension. More fundamentally, however, tai chi teaches people to relax the body instead of tensing in stressful situations. This is a major benefit of partnerwork (see pages 118–119). By repeatedly giving and receiving a push, each partner is offered an opportunity to transform the tension it raises into an alert and dynamic relaxation. With training they discover that a more effective way of dealing with a push is to embrace it rather than deny it. The practice strengthens mental and physical confidence, so that body and mind become reprogramed, reacting with the fight-or-flight response only in moments of real danger. The overall level of tension in the body falls significantly.

Tension in muscles is normal, enabling us to stand and walk. As one group of muscles tenses for action, another relaxes. Normal muscular tension is also beneficial, since in well-exercised legs it will stimulate the upward flow of blood circulating through the veins and lymph flowing along vessels rising from the feet and legs to the heart. The deep veins of the legs send blood flowing upward against the force of gravity to the heart. During exercise, the moving muscles press against the wall of the veins, acting like a pump to speed the blood flow through them. They have the same effect on the lymph vessels.

THE VOLUNTARY MUSCLES

Tai chi is concerned with the muscles we use consciously when we move. These are the voluntary muscles, attached by tendons to the skeleton (right). Tai chi encourages the muscles to work together. This is believed to promote the development of jin, or whole body energy.

THE VOLUNTARY MUSCLES

A tai chi posture, such as Golden Rooster Stands on One Leg (illustrated here) involves almost all the body's voluntary muscles.

Trapezius: *This muscles raises and rotates the shoulder blade and draws the head back or to the side.*

Deltoid: *These cover the shoulder joint and raise and rotate the arm.*

Serratus anterior: *This muscle moves the shoulder blade forward, and assists in arm-raising and pushing.*

Latissimus dorsi: *These large back muscles draw the arms into the chest, extend them and are important in deep breathing.*

Triceps: *These muscles straighten the forearms.*

External oblique: *The muscles at either side of the abdomen that hold the abdomen firm.*

Gluteus maximus: *The gluteals are the large muscles of the buttocks. They raise the body from a stoop and they rotate the thighs.*

Hamstring muscles: *These run from the pelvis to join the tibia just below the knee. They bend the knee and rotate it outward.*

Soleus: *This powerful muscle plays an important part in bending the ankle and pointing the foot.*

Achilles tendon: *The body's strongest tendon, it connects the calf muscle and the ankle.*

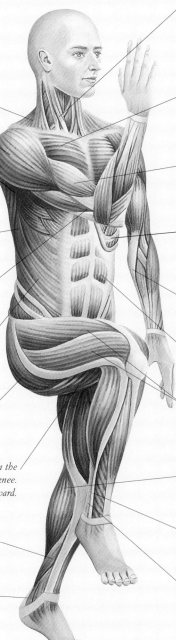

Sternomastoid: *Two neck muscles that independently incline the head toward the shoulder and rotate it left or right, and together help keep the head upright.*

Pectorals: *The large muscles stretching across the chest. They control the shoulder blades and move the arms forward and down.*

Biceps brachi: *Descending from the shoulder to the forearm, the biceps bend the arms at the elbows and help turn the palms upward.*

Intercostal muscles *These small muscles between the ribs help to expand the rib cage on an in-breath and contract it on an out-breath.*

Brachioradialis: *This muscles works with other muscles to turn the palm of the hand upward.*

Rectus abdominis: *Two abdominal muscles that bend the trunk forward or to the side.*

Quadriceps: *A major group of thigh muscles that help raise the leg from the hip, and in a standing position straighten the leg and lock it.*

Gastrocnemius: *The calf muscles have a role in bending the knee and in walking.*

Peronius longus: *These muscles flex or bend the ankle joints.*

Flexor digitorum longus: *Responsible for extending the great toe, one of a group of muscles that are connected to the tibia.*

Body Alignment

ONE OF THE *first benefits of tai chi is a rapid and noticeable improvement in basic posture.*
Tai chi encourages students to key into the natural design of the body. It restores an awareness
of alignments that enable the frame to function with greater ease and strength. Most children
enjoy a natural relationship with the body, but as they grow up, some lose this freedom and
begin to move awkwardly, or gradually forget how to move in a natural and unrestricted way.
Exploring body mechanics helps mind and body to regain some of these lost abilities.

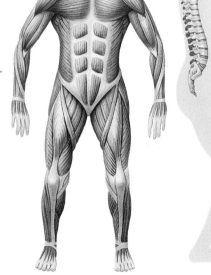

The body is flexible and mobile. Its frame is designed to enable it to sit, lie, stand, walk, run, jump, lift, and carry, and its postural alignment enables the body to perform its movements in a dynamic relationship with gravity.

The human frame is the structural system of skeleton, tendons, ligaments, and muscles, which give the body its shape and alignment when moving or still. The frame is not inert like the frame of a building, but kinetic. Each bone has its correct position in the skeleton, a certain range of movement, and a specific alignment with its neighboring bones, the tendons and ligaments that hold it in place, and the muscles that make its movement possible. The body works as a whole, so the misalignment of bones affects posture and movement.

Stooping and slumping, lifting heavy weights with the body wrongly aligned, aggressive

exercise, and tension all affect the body's frame. Years of such misuse can undermine its alignment, and this can result in back pain, headaches or migraines, and malfunctioning joints. However, the malfunctions that are caused by poor posture can be prevented and eased by realignment through tai chi.

Tai chi works with gravity, allowing it to anchor the body into the earth, working to restore the frame's natural flexibility. It achieves this by relaxing muscles and releasing tension all over the body, allowing bones to resume their intended alignment relative to one another. Many people who learn tai chi feel a sense of strength that comes from having restored the body's natural relationship with gravity and from the fact that bones and muscles that are correctly aligned can be exercised more effectively.

LEFT *The spine is an excellent example of the body working as a holistic system. Its 33 bones or vertebrae are aligned in an s-shape and its two flexible curves, combined with the ability of the vertebrae to work separately yet together at the same time, give the back its marvelous mobility.*

FAR LEFT *Incorrect alignment of the frame – the bones, joints, and muscles – can lead to structural problems such as slipped disks, back pain, and malfunctions of the joints. Tai chi teaches body awareness, so that good posture when lying, sitting, standing, and moving becomes natural.*

STANDING LIKE A MOUNTAIN BETWEEN HEAVEN AND EARTH

This exercise aims to raise awareness of the body's physical support system, and of the relationship between the parts of the body and their alignment, from the feet on the earth to the head in the sky. The thighs and pelvis meet at the hip joint, the largest in the body. Your hip joints are being asked to "soften" and to open up or gently stretch. Your knees are sensitive to alignment. They act as channels, allowing the force of gravity to pass through. The position of the feet affects the alignment of the frame, which rises from them; and from them descends an imaginary channel that anchors the body to the earth center. Become aware of the relationship between your feet and legs and your upper body.

1 Stand comfortably with your feet well apart. Notice how and where the weight of your body comes down though your feet. Is it toward the toes or the heels, the instep or the outside of each foot, or somewhere in the middle?

2 Rock your weight slowly forward to the front of your feet and bring it back. Repeat two more times. When you stop, allow your feet to meet the earth fully, the weight evenly balanced.

3 Bring your weight to the instep. You immediately feel unwanted strain on your knees. They are misaligned and not designed to work properly in this position. Redistribute your weight evenly across your feet.

4 Realign your knees so they follow the direction of the feet. This maintains the correct relationship between the feet, the knees, and the hips. Feel it by dropping your spine a few inches. Look down to see that your kneecap follows the direction of the toes.

5 Stand upright again. Turn your feet to point slightly outward, and once again drop your spine and bend your knees. Check that your knees are in line with your toes. Notice the effect on your hips when doing this.

6 Keeping your legs and upper body still, rock your pelvis backward and forward, then from side to side. Feel your pelvis floating. Circle it a few times in each direction. The pelvic girdle is basin-shaped, a holder and carrier. Feel the link between your lower pelvis and your hip joints, and the relationship between your pelvis and your feet.

7 Dropping the spine and bending the knees softens and opens the hips. Repeat this movement a few times, allowing your hips to move and open. Feel the connection between feet, knees, and hips. Your feet are anchored to give you stability; your hips allow mobility. Now return your feet to parallel.

8 With your feet planted on the ground, your weight distributed evenly so your knees and toes are aligned, and your pelvis free to move, feel how the spine carries you up through your neck toward the sky. Drop your spine to sit into the earth, relax your muscles downward (yin) and simultaneously feel the upward and outward support of your bones (yang).

9 Lift your arms out a little way away from your body. Imagine your shoulder joints open, letting in space. Feel your arms lift farther out. Explore the movement possibilities of your elbows, then your wrists, then turn your fingertips toward each other. Imagine your arms are growing out from your spine, and make a connection between your fingers.

10 Direct your attention to the top of your head. Soften the muscles here and downward through your body. At the same time imagine the bones of your spine lifting you to this point. Feel the polarity between your feet in the earth and your head in the sky. This keeps your spine open or stretched up and down, so that it falls into its natural curved shape.

Stability and Mobility

HERE, WITH THE HELP *of two guided exercises, you can develop a practical understanding of the qualities of stability and mobility. Let your feet meet the earth. Let your knees follow the direction of your toes. Soften your hips. Let your pelvis float and your spine anchor you in the earth and carry you to the sky. These injunctions are the basis of stability and the key to understanding the nature of tai chi movement, for the body's relationship to the earth is like that of an underwater plant, which is anchored to a rock yet moves with ease in the current.*

Many people who begin tai chi are not used to maintaining a low center of gravity, or to using their legs so much. Aching legs are a sign that tai chi is gradually strengthening the limbs. The process works in two ways, so it is through the movements that a beginner develops stability. Trying to deepen the stance by dropping the spine while moving accustoms the legs to work harder and makes it possible to achieve a still lower center of gravity.

This exercise in stability begins with the principles expressed in the posture Stand Like A Mountain Between Heaven and Earth (page 25). It ensures every stance or movement is rooted to the earth, but reaches up to the heavens.

STABILITY

This is a two-person exercise, although the role of your partner is to act as an assistant. Ask your partner to build up the pressure very gradually as you learn to deal with it. Before you begin, find the position Stand Like a Mountain Between Heaven and Earth, and take a moment to relax into it.

1 *When you are feeling comfortably stable and your body has a sense of wholeness, ask your friend to lean in toward you from the side, gently and slowly.*

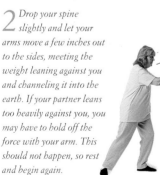

3 *As you become familiar with the feeling of the weight of another body leaning into you from the side and channeling down through your body, ask your friend to roll around you slowly and lean into you from different angles. Notice how you have to make slight changes to your frame to adjust to pressure from different angles.*

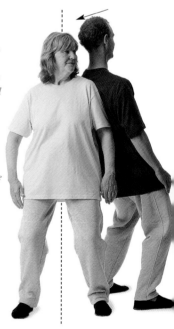

2 *Drop your spine slightly and let your arms move a few inches out to the sides, meeting the weight leaning against you and channeling it into the earth. If your partner leans too heavily against you, you may have to hold off the force with your arm. This should not happen, so rest and begin again.*

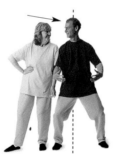

4 *Remain solidly stable as your partner turns while orbiting around you.*

MOBILITY

For this exercise you need a safe, comfortable space to move in, and a blindfold. Play some of your favorite, soothing music. While doing this exercise you will be blindfolded, so you will not be able to read these directions at the same time. Rather than try to memorize them, record yourself reading them or ask a friend to read them out to you. Take your time with this exercise. It will probably last 10 to 20 minutes, but there is no time limit. You may find yourself drawn into the meditation for as long as an hour.

1 Stand, blindfolded, imagining you hold a ball of light in your hands. Play with it for a minute. Now imagine the light pouring from the ball into your hands and wrists. Imagine the light soothing and oiling the joints, and massaging your hands and wrists.

2 Invite the light to move up through your arm bones into your elbows, bringing them freedom of movement. Feel the folding, unfolding, and turning movements of this complex joint, and its link to wrists and hands.

3 Follow the light up your arms and pouring into your shoulder joints. Move your arms forward and back, up and down, and out to the sides, exploring their mobility. Think about how each limb is connected from shoulder to finger joint.

4 Feel the light flood from your shoulder joint into your shoulder blades and move to your neck. Relaxing your face and jaw, move your neck in every direction. Then follow the light as it moves up into your jaw and skull. Explore the movement of your jawbone.

5 The light slowly descends your spine, filling each vertebra and spreading along each rib. Explore the movement possibilities of your upper body. Follow the light down to the sacrum and coccyx. As it circles the pelvic girdle, your hips join the dance. Let yourself move intuitively and creatively.

6 Let the light pour into your hip joints, directing your attention to them and supporting their movement. Listen to your pelvis and follow the knowledge that resides in it.

7 Follow the light down each thighbone. Your knees fill with light. It pours down your shin bones to your ankles and feet. Your whole frame is alight and alive, a dancing skeleton.

8 Bring your body to rest. You may feel like standing or sitting, crouching, squatting, crawling, or even rolling on the floor. Notice your mobility as you move into these different positions. Finish by resting in any position for at least one minute. Remove your blindfold.

Body Shape and Posture

THE QUALITIES OF *stability and mobility work with perfect synchronicity in the tai chi postures, which combine correct body shape with freedom of movement. The result is a solid strength and flexibility. Tai chi is a holistic practice, so all parts of the body – hips and heels, pelvis and spine, shoulders and hands – work as one.*

The shape adopted by the body in the tai chi stance encourages the release of stress expressed in the shoulders by relaxing and opening the joints, and the muscles that make them work, restoring the natural flow of energy around the arms and head.

The spine effects the turn, which gives the changing shapes their spirals and circles. Turning massages the internal organs and enlivens the basic posture. The vertebrae work together to turn the body from the sacrum upward.

The sacrum transfers the body's weight from the spine to the pelvis, and via the hip joints to the legs, ankles, and feet. The hip joints need to be soft (relaxed), open, and free to move, so the legs, knees, ankles, and feet are aligned.

The pelvis should be held without tension, as if it were floating, and in its natural position. It should not be pushed right forward nor tilted unnaturally back.

The knees follow the direction of the feet and never lock straight. When the body weight is seated mainly in the back leg, the front knee stays slightly bent. When the weight is mainly forward, the back knee is unlocked, though the back leg is extended.

Always keep the head erect and maintain a link between spine, head, and sky.

Complete freedom of movement is given to the elbow joint to allow the forearm and hand full creative expression, with minimal change occurring in the upper arm and shoulders. The elbow joint therefore needs to be kept relaxed and open to facilitate the flow of energy to the wrist and hand.

A push may appear to be a movement of the hands, but it is part of a movement that begins with the feet and is transmitted via the legs and spine to the arms and hands.

The hands may be held in line with the forearms or pulled up and back, but should not droop from the wrists. In some postures, keeping the wrists in line with the forearms enables the elbows to find their correct place.

While the upper body weaves, spirals, and circles, the legs and feet must remain correctly aligned to maintain stability.

The ankle joints become more flexible with practice. The semi-sitting stance exercises the ankles, stimulating the flow of energy along the legs to the feet.

The feet must be sensitive, alert, and comfortably anchored to the ground when the body weight is forward, when it is back, and while it is moving from back to front or front to back.

THE BASIC STANCE

Although every tai chi posture is carried out while standing, the characteristic stance, shown left, is rather like standing and sitting at the same time. By techniques such as keeping the feet firmly planted on the ground, keeping the knees flexible and never locking them, and dropping the spine, you sit yourself into a stance, and maintain this basic posture while moving. This illustration analyzes the basic tai chi stance, and the guidelines given apply to all the postures. Practice the stance as a static posture often, until you are confident enough to be able to adopt it without practice.

ALIGNING THE HANDS

The following exercise demonstrates the difference between aligning the hands with the forearms and letting them hang down from the wrists.

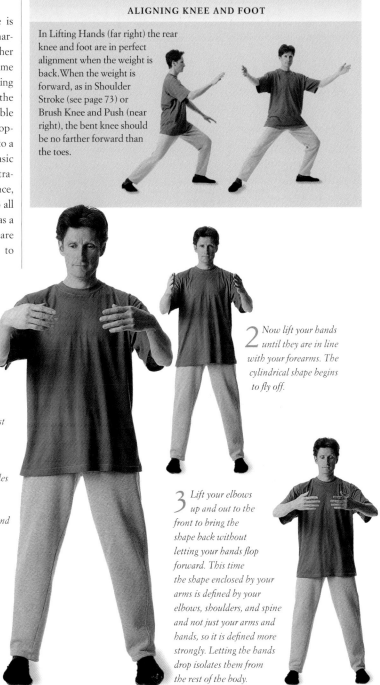

ALIGNING KNEE AND FOOT

In Lifting Hands (far right) the rear knee and foot are in perfect alignment when the weight is back. When the weight is forward, as in Shoulder Stroke (see page 73) or Brush Knee and Push (near right), the bent knee should be no farther forward than the toes.

1 *Stand with your arms lifted to chest level and the palms of your hands facing you with the fingertips spread about 2 inches apart from each other. Let your elbows hang close to your sides and your wrists go limp so that your hands drop. Imagine your arms and hands are enclosing something large and cylindrical against your chest.*

2 *Now lift your hands until they are in line with your forearms. The cylindrical shape begins to fly off.*

3 *Lift your elbows up and out to the front to bring the shape back without letting your hands flop forward. This time the shape enclosed by your arms is defined by your elbows, shoulders, and spine and not just your arms and hands, so it is defined more strongly. Letting the hands drop isolates them from the rest of the body.*

Inside the Body

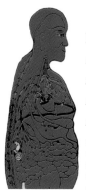

BY COMPARISON WITH *the efficient internal organization of the body, the way most people run their external lives seems chaotic. The perfectly regulated systems that keep the body alive give their unceasing best from the moment of conception to the time of death. Tai chi offers its steady, rhythmic movements as a link between the two. It acknowledges that we are at all times spirit, mind, emotion, and*

LEFT *Traditional Chinese medicine recognizes the importance of the kidneys to health, as this illustration of the internal organs shows.*

physique. And it reinforces the role of the body's internal systems by supporting the working of all its organs, from outer skin to heart and brain deep in its interior.

Although the body's organs function with scarcely an interruption whether the rest of the body is sick or healthy, tense or relaxed, the quality of their functioning fluctuates in ways that often go unnoticed. The health of an organ depends on a network of mental, emotional, and physical conditions. Someone who is feeling good, fulfilled, and wanted by other people will be likely to have well-functioning organs, and, if that person also exercises and follows a healthy diet, excellent health.

Studies show that the body works best when the mind is content, but we have known this instinctively for centuries. Throughout history and across cultural boundaries the liver has been associated with the emotion of anger. Bile, crucial to the breakdown of fats (see pages 34–35), is abundantly produced by the liver when a person is happy. This sensitive organ reduces its bile production in response to anger.

RELEASE THROUGH TAI CHI

Any tai chi exercise can work toward release of tension, anger, or other pent-up emotions. The third preparatory exercise, the Rainbow Circle (see page 58), for example, focuses on healing the kidneys. The following exercise is helpful for releasing emotion. It also massages the kidneys and loosens tightness and feelings of rigidity in the spine. Adopt any strong tai chi stance and relax as deeply as you can. Lift your arms as high as you like and turn your body from one side to the other quite vigorously. At the completion of each turn stop suddenly and shout HEY! or SHOO! Feel the release coming through your arms and out of your fingers.

Through regular daily practice and especially through partner practice, tai chi teaches new ways of dealing with anger and

other strong emotion. It teaches techniques of self-expression as the best way of achieving this (see pages 124–131). It is well known that depression can be the result of pent-up anger, and that anger can result from frustration. These emotions must be allowed to flow rather than be blocked. The flow may be generated through speaking, for example, or writing, or painting.

The delicate, intricate kidneys filter about 15 gallons of water and waste products from the blood each day, releasing about 3 pints as urine. They eliminate poisons such as nicotine, and metals, such as mercury and lead (see pages 34–35). According to Traditional Chinese Medicine, the kidneys store life-essence or jing. The adrenal glands, which produce the hormone adrenaline, sit on top of the kidneys, so these organs are associated with fear. This, in turn, is related to willpower. Feelings of timidity can lead to a holding back from life. Working with a tai chi partner is an excellent antidote to timidity.

SHALLOW BREATHING

Breathing is normally powered by the diaphragm, a large, dome-shaped muscle that separates the chest from the abdomen. Its rhythmic movements enable you to draw in as many as 20,000 breaths and 5,000 gallons (500 bushells) of air in a day. If you are in a state of anxiety or depression, however, you do not make use of the diaphragm and other muscles of the lower chest. Breathing takes place mainly in the top part of the chest, and the amount of air you take in is much reduced, so that the body is starved of oxygen and chi, or life energy.

Shallow breathing due to anxiety and tension is a growing problem in modern Western countries. As well as exacerbating imbalances of the mind, such as depression, it undermines health. Not enough oxygen dissolves from the lungs into the bloodstream (see page 39), and to remain healthy all body tissues need a regular supply of oxygen

from the blood. In stressful situations the speed and depth of breathing change, and the natural, cyclical rhythm of breathing is lost. People hold their breath in fear.

Poor breathing means low energy levels, because along with oxygen, the blood supplies the tissues with nutrients (see pages 32–33). Attempts to raise energy levels by eating more can have the same effect as overloading a choked fire with more wood. What is needed is a reshaping of the fuel, so that more oxygen and nutrients can reach the body's cells. Tai chi works to restore the habit of natural, deep breathing, to enable the body to release energy most efficiently from the available fuel – the circulating blood. The workings of the body are interconnected, and the quality of the blood depends on the well-being of the vital organs, the health of which is shaped in turn by the quality of the blood they receive.

BREATHING IN

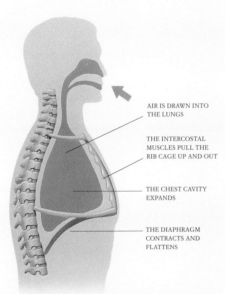

AIR IS DRAWN INTO
THE LUNGS

THE INTERCOSTAL
MUSCLES PULL THE
RIB CAGE UP AND OUT

THE CHEST CAVITY
EXPANDS

THE DIAPHRAGM
CONTRACTS AND
FLATTENS

BREATHING OUT

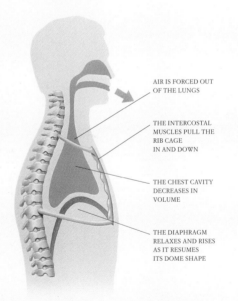

AIR IS FORCED OUT
OF THE LUNGS

THE INTERCOSTAL
MUSCLES PULL THE
RIB CAGE
IN AND DOWN

THE CHEST CAVITY
DECREASES IN
VOLUME

THE DIAPHRAGM
RELAXES AND RISES
AS IT RESUMES
ITS DOME SHAPE

Tai chi works holistically to improve the functioning of body and mind. It acknowledges emotions as part of the human condition, and as a way of airing them, creating a space in which they can begin to dissolve, opening the way to a happier state. Just as massage can release nervous tension, tai chi can dislodge emotion, superficial or deep-seated, held in the body. Any tai chi exercise can work toward release of tension, anger, or other pent-up emotions. When this happens in practice, it can disrupt a seemingly harmonious state, but having cleared away an emotional block, the body will function better.

The Circulation

TAI CHI PROVIDES the exercise the body needs to maintain its marvelous circulatory systems. First, it stimulates the pumping action of the heart. For many people, an over-sedentary lifestyle results in sluggish circulation of the blood and of the lymph fluid, which supplies the tissues with water and nutrients. Tai chi exercise combined with regular massage provide the necessary stimulants to both.

All the cells in the body are bathed in watery tissue fluid in which are dissolved the nutrients they need to live. Tissue fluid circulates in the bloodstream. The pumping action of the heart channels blood along arteries into a network of ever smaller blood vessels down to the capillaries, the smallest blood vessels that reach from the organs deep inside the body to the skin.

Molecules of tissue fluid containing water, oxygen, and essential nutrients can pass through the capillary walls into the minute spaces between the cells. From there they can be absorbed when needed by the surrounding cells.

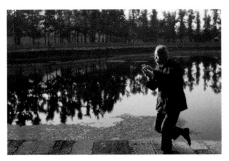

ABOVE *Muscular tension in well-exercised legs stimulates the return of circulating blood and lymph upward to the heart.*

All the time, cells excrete excess water and unwanted chemicals such as carbon dioxide through their walls back into the tissue fluid, which drains into the bloodstream through tiny veins called venules. But a proportion of it, along with waste products such as dead cells and bacteria, becomes lymph, a milky fluid mixed with white blood cells, fats from ducts in the intestine, and proteins. Lymph is filtered through lymph nodes packed with disease-fighting lymphocytes or white blood cells.

The channels that transport lymph from the tissues back to join the bloodstream have no pump. One-way valves in lymph vessels ensure the fluid circulates in the right direction and the pumping action of muscles during exercise keep the lymph circulating.

Tai chi practice maintains a healthy circulation because it uses the body's natural tension to establish a balance between tension and relaxation. As one group of muscles tenses, another relaxes, and this mechanism enables us to walk, stand, and sit, for example. The wonderful synchronicity between heartbeats, breaths, and movements, which we first experienced in our mother's womb, may be rediscovered by relaxing into tai chi practice.

Stress is a nervous stimulus that destroys this synchronicity, and the heart responds by weakening and becoming diseased. It is therapeutic to shine a light into the dark corners of the heart, simply by listening to it. Take the time to be still and quiet – after tai chi practice is ideal because body and mind are alive, receptive, and responsive.

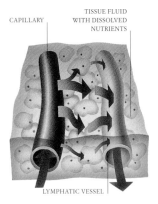

CAPILLARY

TISSUE FLUID WITH DISSOLVED NUTRIENTS

LYMPHATIC VESSEL

LEFT *Tissue fluid containing water, dissolved oxygen, and nutrients such as calcium and glucose passes through the capillary walls to bathe every cell in the body.*

BLOOD AND LYMPH CIRCULATION

Tissue fluid, which nourishes the body's cells, is circulated through the bloodstream by the pumping of the heart. Arteries, veins, blood vessels and capillaries are the network that carry blood to all parts of the body. The lymphatic system (below) is an essential part of the body's immune system. Lymphocytes, which fight infection, are carried through the lymph vessels.

The carotid arteries branch from the subclavian arteries to supply the head with blood.

The subclavian arteries branch directly from the aorta and supply the arteries of the arm.

The jugular veins collect blood returning from the head and channel it into the superior vena cava and the heart.

The pulmonary artery takes blood from the right side of the heart to be oxygenated by the lungs.

The two pulmonary veins carry oxygenated blood, transporting it from the lungs back to the heart.

The inferior vena cava is a major vein. It collects deoxygenated blood from the abdomen and legs and returns it to the right atrium of the heart.

Most arteries in the arms have more than one vein running alongside, so that warm blood returns to the heart even when the hands are cold.

The aorta, the largest artery, receives oxygenated blood pumped from the left ventricle of the heart and carries it to the arteries serving the head, limbs, and major organs.

The femoral vein carries blood from the leg, upward to the trunk.

Tonsils are masses of tissue in the throat packed with lymphocytes that attack cancer cells and microorganisms.

Thymus gland Until the teen years this gland is an important producer of lymphocytes.

The radial artery carries blood from the arm to the hand. At the point where it crosses the wrist a pulse can be felt.

The armpit is the site of many lymph nodes, which filter harmful cells and organisms from the lymph.

Thoracic ducts These vessels carry lymph from the abdomen to the neck, where they return it to the bloodstream by emptying it into a large vein near the heart.

The femoral arteries distribute blood from the aorta to the thighs and branch to supply the lower legs.

The great saphenous vein runs from the foot up the inside of the leg almost to the hip, and is the longest vein.

Lymphatic vessels drain the body tissues of excess fluid and waste products, and transport them to the lymph nodes to be filtered.

The spleen produces lymphocytes and releases them into the lymph vessels.

Small deep veins in the legs lie close to arteries, so cold blood from the feet is warmed on its way back to the heart.

Digestion and Elimination

THE ENERGY FOR *body maintenance, growth, and repair comes from the food we ingest and transport to nourish every part of the body down to its smallest component, the cell. An important part of this complex system involves eliminating the waste products secreted by the cells. The organs of the digestive and excretory systems fit into the protective cavities provided by the ribs and the pelvic girdle*

LEFT *Needles at Sea Bottom improves digestion by massaging the colon.*

– all but one, the largest, which covers the body from head to toe and is its first line of defense against disease: the skin.

Soft and extraordinarily flexible, yet a strong supporting structure and an almost impenetrable barrier against invasion by microorganisms, the skin is a key member of the team of major organs that regulate the body's water balance. It does this through sweating. It works with the intestine, the kidneys, the lungs, and the colon to balance the quantity of water taken in with the amount leaving the body, and this critical balance scarcely deviates from an astonishingly narrow margin, whatever sudden changes in temperature or extra intake of food and drink the body may have to deal with. When

the organs of digestion break down the food we eat into their basic molecules, they are absorbed into the blood and the water balance ensures that nutrients needed by the cells reach them.

Digestion changes the food we eat into usable energy for body maintenance, growth, and repair. Digestion begins with the sensation of hunger and the stimulation of the salivary glands in the mouth. The brain sensitizes the stomach to good news about food, encouraging its digestive abilities. The best way to look after the stomach is to eat with enjoyment and dedication.

From gullet (esophagus) to colon, the entire digestive system is governed by rhythmic contractions, called peristalsis, of the muscular walls of organs such as the stomach and intestines. The colon (large intestine) is especially susceptible to disturbances of its natural rhythm, which cause complaints such as irritable bowel syndrome (IBS), in which the colon is affected by spasms. In particular, exercises and postures that involve squatting massage the colon directly, encouraging normal peristaltic movements. Similarly, with the repeated turning of the spine in tai chi postures, the kidneys, a delicate organism of fundamental importance to the body's health, receive a continual massage.

Digestion is a complex process that is strongly influenced by emotions. Appetite loss is often an early sign of emotional disturbance. Tai chi relieves the stress that can have a catastrophic effect on the harmonious working of these bodily processes. Its generally calming influence on the body encourages the organs of digestion and elimination to function normally.

THE SKIN

The skin regulates the body's water balance by sweating. Each day large quantities of water containing traces of salt and other chemicals are excreted through the sweat glands buried deep in the skin. The steady build up of heat generated through tai chi exercise opens the pores of the skin, assisting this eliminative process. Sweat on the skin surface cools the body when it is too hot.

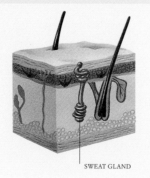

SWEAT GLAND

DIGESTION

Digestion begins as food enters the mouth, where the process of breakdown starts. Digestion is both a physical and a chemical process in that the food is cut up by the teeth and churned by the stomach and the muscular movements of the gut. At the same time, however, it is broken down by chemicals released at different stages in the digestive process.

In addition to the frontline organs of digestion, illustrated here – the stomach, liver, and small intestine – the lungs play an indirect role in digestion. By supplying oxygen, they allow the fire of the digestive system to burn and so release energy. Along with the colon and kidneys, they also have a role in elimination and in maintaining the body's water balance, since water vapor is released with every out-breath.

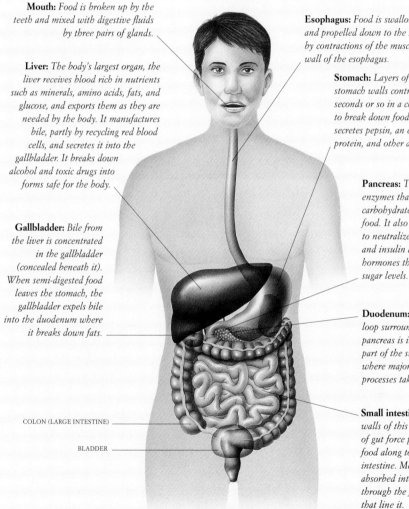

Mouth: *Food is broken up by the teeth and mixed with digestive fluids by three pairs of glands.*

Liver: *The body's largest organ, the liver receives blood rich in nutrients such as minerals, amino acids, fats, and glucose, and exports them as they are needed by the body. It manufactures bile, partly by recycling red blood cells, and secretes it into the gallbladder. It breaks down alcohol and toxic drugs into forms safe for the body.*

Gallbladder: *Bile from the liver is concentrated in the gallbladder (concealed beneath it). When semi-digested food leaves the stomach, the gallbladder expels bile into the duodenum where it breaks down fats.*

COLON (LARGE INTESTINE)

BLADDER

Esophagus: *Food is swallowed and propelled down to the stomach by contractions of the muscular wall of the esophagus.*

Stomach: *Layers of muscle in the stomach walls contract every 20 seconds or so in a churning motion to break down food. The stomach secretes pepsin, an enzyme to digest protein, and other digestive juices.*

Pancreas: *This gland secretes enzymes that digest proteins, carbohydrates, fats, and other food. It also secretes chemicals to neutralize stomach acids, and insulin and glucagon, hormones that regulate blood-sugar levels.*

Duodenum: *This C-shaped loop surrounding the pancreas is in fact the first part of the small intestine, where major digestive processes take place.*

Small intestine: *The muscular walls of this 21-foot length of gut force partially digested food along to the large intestine. Meanwhile it is absorbed into the blood through the fingerlike villi that line it.*

EALING TERTIARY COLLEGE
LEARNING RESOURCE CENTRE - EALING GREEN

Sensory Systems

TAI CHI PRACTICE has the effect of heightening awareness. This process begins with the body, because discovering how and why the body moves raises the consciousness. Developing new ways of responding to other people as a result of learning partner practice expands the awareness. And as tai chi encourages the exploration of the relationship between the self and the cosmos, there is the potential for the awareness to reach new heights.

Tai chi is a sensual practice; learning it involves expanding sensory awareness, which is rooted in the brain. The cerebellum, an older part of the brain that forms a small sub-brain below the larger and more highly developed cerebrum, coordinates the body's posture, balance, and fine voluntary movements. Studying tai chi stimulates this area of the brain. It also brings increased sensitivity through developing the quality of touch, particularly in the partner exercises. Each person learns to listen, through touch, to the other. The learning process extends naturally to include the thoughts and feelings of the partner. The hands, which have more nerve endings than any other part of the body, gather information. Each partner is encouraged to feel more deeply, to extend awareness through touch toward the other person. In time they learn to read the moment when a partner's push is about to begin, or choose the best moment to release a push.

Through partner practice it should become apparent that too much reliance tends to be placed on the sense of sight. In Asia, blind people train as masseurs, their sense of touch being especially keen. Sighted people realize how much they rely on vision when they practice while blindfolded.

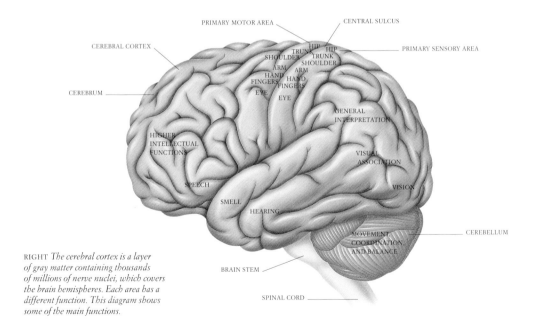

RIGHT *The cerebral cortex is a layer of gray matter containing thousands of millions of nerve nuclei, which covers the brain hemispheres. Each area has a different function. This diagram shows some of the main functions.*

CEREBELLUM

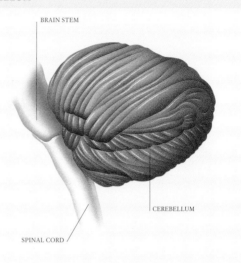

BRAIN STEM

CEREBELLUM

SPINAL CORD

The organs of balance in the ear send information about posture to the cerebellum. It is positioned behind the brain stem, the oldest part of the brain, and connected to it by nerve pathways that supply data from structures involved in movement. The tendons, for example, send information about the state of tension or relaxation of the muscles, and the cerebellum controls muscle tone, always keeping one-third of muscle fibers contracted. The cerebellum is called the "small brain" because it lies beneath the much larger cerebrum, the most evolved brain area where higher brain functions take place. It communicates with areas in the cerebrum that control movement. The cerebellum coordinates the information it receives and modifies the signals sent to the muscles to ensure movements are smoothly coordinated. It controls balance, working on an automatic level so that we sit, stand, or lean without having to think about how to do it. The cerebellum is capable of learning, so that although tai chi movements may be difficult at first, with practice the cerebellum learns their patterns and incorporates them on a semi-conscious level.

Tai chi training works to establish a healthy balance between seeing and feeling. To do this it is essential to dissolve the need for precise, focused vision and allow peripheral vision to come alive. The eye always follows movement, and tai chi utilizes this mechanism by encouraging peripheral vision. Looking straight ahead and focusing on a single object transforms the object into a complete experience. Withdrawing the attention from it slightly allows the consciousness to expand, to include a larger dimension so that although the eye continues to look forward, the mind becomes aware of the shape and feeling of the space either side, and any movement in that space becomes evident.

Spatial awareness is a survival mechanism, an ability that develops from infancy. Tai chi extends and develops it. In time, people become acutely aware of their personal space and develop a sensitivity to the boundaries of other people's space. This heightened awareness naturally extends into the emotions. People often find they can assess the atmosphere of a room, a person, a building, or a landscape more quickly.

THE SENSE OF SMELL

This sense is a powerful force in human consciousness, essential to our survival. People talk about scenting fear or danger. We have a long memory for smells, and a smell remembered from childhood can evoke deep feelings. Becoming sensitive to smells is a way of extending the consciousness, but. awareness of this sense tends to be masked by the overdominance of sight, hearing, speech, and touch. To bring it to the forefront, the influence of the other senses needs to be reduced. In partner practice, for example, you might use your sense of smell as a possible extra source of information. Through exercises like this you raise your general awareness and sensitivity.

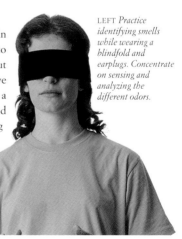

LEFT *Practice identifying smells while wearing a blindfold and earplugs. Concentrate on sensing and analyzing the different odors.*

Breathing

THE WORD "CHI" *is sometimes translated as "breath" since breathing is so closely associated with the energy of life. It is said that the spirit enters the body of a child the moment it takes its first breath. The physical links between breathing and life are clear. Tai chi encourages the development of a naturally deep pattern of breathing in which the rhythm of the breath is synchronized with the flow of the movements. This is whole breathing, and its aim is to reap the countless benefits a dynamic metabolism can bring to mind and body.*

The breath connects the inner life of the body to the outside world through the lungs, which are carrying on a moment-by-moment dialog between the body and the space it inhabits. The breath is a messenger, carrying one message into the body and sending a different one to the outside world. This message is carried on the air, which fills the outside world, is drawn temporarily into the body, and expelled from it in an altered form. Air is the element associated with the astrological sign Gemini, the ruling planet of which is Mercury, the messenger. If the rhythm of the breathing is even, the message carried on the expelled air is one of harmony. Alternatively, sound may surf the out-breath and travel through the air as messages in speech. Air drawn into the body is needed

RIGHT *When moving back in Push posture, some teachers advise breathing out, and breathing in on the forward step. Experiment to find the best way for you.*

for its oxygen, the gift of green plants to the global atmosphere, donated over billions of years and now under severe threat from the destructive aspects of modern living.

Breathing is an unconscious process, controlled by the respiration center in the brain. It is impossible to stop yourself breathing long enough to endanger your life. However, some aspects of breathing, such as the speed and depth of the breath, are under voluntary control. Because of the importance of breathing to well-being, many health systems seek to develop techniques for improving breathing, such as yoga, and the Chinese systems of neigung and qigung. Tai chi emphasizes natural breathing.

Everything in nature, from the tides to the seasons, is cyclical, and breathing is one of life's many cycles with its own natural rhythm. Through harmonious, rhythmic movement tai chi harmonizes the rhythm of the breath with that of

the body's movements. It comes through regular practice, but when it happens, a doorway opens and the whole organization of the body changes. It is as if each cell begins to relax and enjoy life, moment by moment, as if body, mind, and soul are able to rest. This resting gives the body a chance to heal, to draw in the vital energy whose circulation through the body we block through repeated episodes of anxiety.

However, there are different theories on how to breathe correctly in tai chi. Some say the postures should end on an out-breath, with the moves between postures being executed on an in-breath. This makes sense in a posture such as Push (see page 69), when the outward movement of the breath complements the outward impetus of the posture. Others argue the opposite, that the in-breath is the energy that fills the posture. The internal expansion in a posture such as Ward Off (see pages 66–67) supports the argument, so this posture, the argument goes, should begin on an out-breath and end on an in-breath.

Do not let the issue become a source of anxiety, which can inhibit

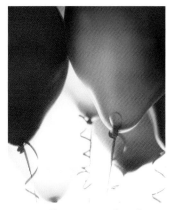

ABOVE *Close your eyes and visualize a bunch of colorful balloons. Choose the brightest, and imagine the touch of the balloon's surface against your skin as your hands squeeze its pliable surface.*

healthy breathing. The best advice is to experiment with different ways of breathing in a personal search for harmony of movement and breathing.

THE PULSE OF THE BREATH

This exercise is aimed at developing sensitivity. It is simple, but you may at first find it hard to focus. With practice stronger feeling develops in your hands. Allow five minutes.

Sit or stand comfortably upright. Lift your hands to face each other about 18 inches apart. Think of the space between your hands and imagine you hold a balloon. Squeeze it a little, then again several times. Focus on it until you can feel the pressure. Now direct your awareness to your breathing and notice how the pressure between your hands and the balloon's shape changes in relation to your breathing. Is the pressure greatest on an in-breath, an out-breath, or during the brief pause between in and out and in? Does your body feel different when breathing out from breathing in?

THE LUNGS

Each lung looks like a tree with a cluster of grapes at the end of every branching twig. These structures, called alveoli, have walls lined with a thin layer of cells through which molecules of air and water can pass into tiny blood vessels called capillaries surrounding them. With each breath, oxygen from the air you breathe in passes into the blood, and carbon dioxide and other gases pass into the lung along with water vapor to be breathed out into the air.

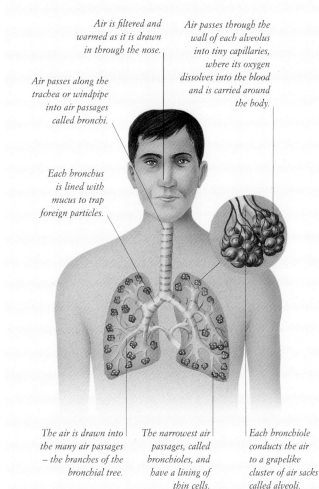

Air is filtered and warmed as it is drawn in through the nose.

Air passes through the wall of each alveolus into tiny capillaries, where its oxygen dissolves into the blood and is carried around the body.

Air passes along the trachea or windpipe into air passages called bronchi.

Each bronchus is lined with mucus to trap foreign particles.

The air is drawn into the many air passages – the branches of the bronchial tree.

The narrowest air passages, called bronchioles, and have a lining of thin cells.

Each bronchiole conducts the air to a grapelike cluster of air sacks called alveoli.

39

The Energy Centers

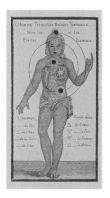

THE IDEA THAT *life energy flows around the body along channels is common to many Eastern medical systems. In Chinese medicine the life force, or chi, flows along channels called meridians; while ancient Hindu medical texts call the energy of life prana, and the channels along which it flows nadis. Spaced along the body's principal nadi, running from the groin along the spine to the head, are seven chakras – vortices of concentrated energy. Chinese medicine also teaches that the body has seven major energy centers – points where the chi is more densely concentrated.*

LEFT *The positions of the chakras, or energy centers, in Hindu medicine corresponds with the major life systems, such as the reproductive system, and with the endocrine glands.*

There is more to the body than its surface physiology. While the many meridians carrying their streams of life energy remain invisible, they can be detected, rather like water holes in the bush, the location of which can be detected by a higher level of activity taking place around them than in the surrounding terrain. They have been identified in almost all Eastern medical systems. Acupuncture, for example, identifies 14 meridians, while the traditional Tibetan healing system recognizes many more. And although the existence of the seven energy centers is as yet unproven scientifically, their location is known to correspond with the plexes – concentrated networks of major nerves, such as the solar plexus just below the diaphragm – and with the positions of the endocrine glands, which secrete hormones.

From the energy centers, the life force travels along the meridians to fill every cell. The body senses any changes taking place in the energy surrounding it, and responds to them, so that changes in the body will be transmitted outward and will affect and to some extent shape the surrounding energy field. Aspects of this energy field, such as the electromagnetic energy generated by all living things, can be measured, but some individuals have the power to see it in its colorful entirety, as an aura emanating from the body.

Tai chi spans the physical, mental, and energetic aspects of life. It shapes and reshapes the body's energy field, keeping its channels clear and energizing them. It opens up exciting possibilities for change to be brought about consciously through working with different aspects of the body. The tai chi postures gather energy and generate it, speed its circulation around the body to make hands and feet glow with warmth, calm its turbulence until the mind rests in tranquility, or send it outward.

It is the potential to regulate the flow of energy that gives tai chi its celebrated healing powers. With a rudimentary knowledge of energy pathways and centers, you can harness the power of movement to unblock emotional energy and ease muscular tension, restore feeling, and heighten awareness. This is why it is not essential to know a great deal about the system of the meridians and energy centers in order to practice tai chi, although for anyone interested it could be a valuable study. Instead, feeling the effects of a posture on your body's meridians and energy centers, and witnessing the effects of the changes it brings about in your energy patterns can enrich your practice and enable you to master your life.

Tai chi acts on the energy centers of the body to stimulate them and to open the mind and body to their influence. There are seven centers, but the higher extension point might be thought of as an eighth. It lies 18 inches above the top of the head, at the top of the aura, or energy field. Each center corresponds with one of the major nerve junctions and with the glands of the endocrine system, which release directly into the blood hormones that affect the bio-rhythms, such as the cycle of sleep and wakefulness.

The word "hormone" comes from a Greek word meaning "urge on." It is the urging of hormones governing the sexual impulses that creates new life, and prompts a mother to begin birthing. Thus, the energy centers form part of an integrated system that includes our

RIGHT *The location of the energy centers is known to correspond with the body's main plexes (junctions of major nerves) and the endocrine glands, which secrete hormones.*

sensitivity, awareness, and behavior. The energy centers are earthed through the root or base chakra in the pelvis and lifted into the dimension of spirit through the crown chakra at the top of the head. In tai chi, earthing is carried out by dropping the pelvis, as if it descended through the legs and feet into the ground; and lifting is effected by raising the top of the head as if it were suspended from above.

Many of the postures in the tai chi form energize one or more of the chakras. The shape made by the body stimulates activity in the energy body. In the posture White Crane Spreads Wings, for instance, one hand is planted down at

the level of the pelvic floor and the other is turned up to the heavens and raised above the head, to link the root and crown chakras. The open shape made by the front of the body energizes the solar plexus, focusing it outward.

This interaction with the energy centers gives practice an exciting dimension. Each center is associated with certain qualities – the heart center, for example, with passion and compassion, envy and love, the throat center with communication and expression. Certain postures might be carried out with the intention of accessing a particular energy center and stimulating the qualities associated with it. If the qualities are in disequilibrium, if, for instance, jealousy is destroying a loving relationship, movements might be carried out to restore a balance. To practice with the awareness of the relationship of tai chi to the body's energy centers provides rich possibilities for self-development.

ACTIVATING THE SECONDARY CENTERS

The tai chi postures continually move all the joints of the body and this activates a system of secondary energy centers, located on the body's major joints: the shoulders and elbows, the hips and the knees, and ankles. There are also centers located on the palm of each hand and in the center of each foot. It is important to focus awareness on these points when practicing. Moving with this awareness is like opening a doorway through which energy can pass and is an especially effective method of self-healing.

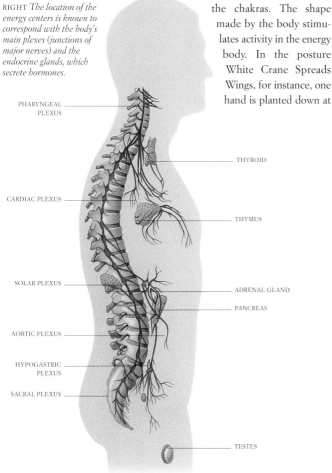

PHARYNGEAL PLEXUS

CARDIAC PLEXUS

SOLAR PLEXUS

AORTIC PLEXUS

HYPOGASTRIC PLEXUS

SACRAL PLEXUS

THYROID

THYMUS

ADRENAL GLAND

PANCREAS

TESTES

41

Preparing for Practice

ABOVE *Choose clothes that are comfortable and do not constrain your mobility. Try to wear natural fibers.*

PRACTICING TAI CHI *stimulates the complicated, interacting system of body and mind. Before beginning the movements it is useful to have an overview of the nature and purpose of tai chi practice. The guidelines outlined here are an introduction to the practicalities of tai chi and a useful reference to be consulted between practice sessions.*

Practice may take place anywhere, indoors or out. Concentration is important, so some people may prefer to practice alone in a quiet place. Bear in mind, however, that in China, where tai chi originated, it is customary to practice outdoors. In towns or the countryside people seek out places – a rooftop or a hilltop, a park or a garden, beneath trees or beside water – where the air is full of chi or life energy.

Tai chi is energizing rather than tiring, and practicing a form for 10 minutes makes a marvelous start to the day. Alternatively, practice can be relaxing after a frenetic day, making sleep more satisfying. It is wise not to practice for an hour immediately after eating a full meal since digestion uses a great deal of energy. Since tai chi also uses energy, however, it is equally important not to practice on an empty stomach. A light snack half hour or so before beginning is advisable.

To be effective, practice needs to be regular. Although it may be impossible to avoid missing a day now and again, aim to practice for 10 minutes a day at first. Most people find their practice sessions gradually lengthen, some lasting as

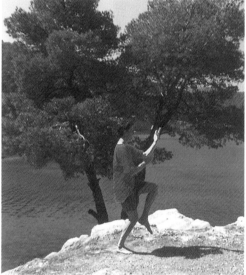

LEFT *More and more Westerners are following the Chinese custom of practicing outdoors where the air is healthiest.*

BELOW *Footwear for tai chi needs to be light and comfortable. The feet, like the rest of the body, should not be restricted during practice.*

long as 90 minutes. Three minutes' heartfelt endeavor is always better, however, than one hour's dutiful drudge. If one cannot be involved mentally as well as physically, it is best to cease practicing and resume when inspiration returns. Invite the earth of the body, the light of the mind, the fire of the passion, and the wisdom of the soul to the feast of each practice.

Try from the beginning to move with focus and intent, not in a heavy, forced manner but with simplicity

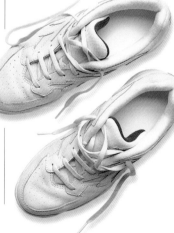

and the light, innocent, inquisitiveness of a child playing in the sand. This will develop a natural coordination of mind and body and the flexibility to continue learning. It is good always to be uncertain as to what each posture, each movement, will bring.

Books about tai chi can be helpful, especially to beginners, and it is wise to listen to a teacher's advice. But most important of all is to check out what they say for yourself. Theoretical knowledge is valuable, but personal knowledge is treasure and students must be careful not to dull the spirit's edge by following theory blindly. It is essential to heed feelings, intuition, and inspiration in search of a personal path. Always ask questions, find out what works and does not work, and why. Never be afraid to improvise around a theme and explore possibilities.

Tai chi practice should be alive. A session may be seen as focused training for living, so qualities that develop there should be taken out into daily life. One might feel like devoting a day to exploring the nature of balance in all aspects of life. Another day it may be listening or spatial awareness. A morning might be spent playing with peripheral vision. At home, at work, or out shopping there is always the potential for letting practice and everyday life become one.

Tai chi is a multidimensional art that can work on all levels of life. It can release the creative side of its practitioners nature, fueling the desire for self-expression through art, drama or other activities (see page 125).

LEARNING TO RELAX

Before moving, spend some time focusing on each part of your body, so that every part of it is relaxed but alert, ready for movement. Start with the feet, where movement is rooted, to be executed from the legs, controlled by the waist, and materialized in the hands and fingers. Work slowly up to the head.

Your head must be upright. Soften the top by relaxing it physically and mentally. Relax your jawbone and imagine that your skull gives space to your brain.

Relax your face, softening your mouth and the area around your eyes. Imagine your face has an open attitude.

Lift your shoulders and drop them to release tension and unwanted uptightness.

Relax your neck.

Relax your elbows so they fall into a natural position.

Starting with your hands and spreading up your arms to your whole body, soften the flesh and muscles away from the bones.

Keep your arms relaxed but alert, always ready to stretch. Imagine your arms growing out from your spine, with space developing in your shoulders, elbows, and wrists.

Soften the chest to let the chi sink to the lower tantien.

Check that your knees follow the direction of your feet, now and during practice.

Let your hip joints move freely. Feel how they can open and close.

Drop the base of your spine into the earth while lifting the upper spine through your neck and your head. Imagine space growing between each vertebra. Imagine your spine opens right across your back and into your arms.

Your feet are the link with the earth on which practice is built. Soften and relax them to allow maximum contact with the ground.

Moves and Postures

ALTHOUGH THE FORM *is the pillar that supports tai chi, the movements are its foundation.*
Yang Lu-chan, founder of the classic Yang-style tai chi who lived during the 1700s,
simply taught a repertoire of moves and postures that he adapted to individual students' needs.
The form, though central to modern tai chi, has evolved only during the last 200 to 300 years.
Today as in the past, the principles of movement are the heart of tai chi practice.

The form is an unbroken succession of movements in which all parts of the body, from the crown of the head, the face and the eyes, to the fingers and toes move in harmony. There is no one definitive form, and the movements practiced differ from tai chi style to style. In the classic Yang form, for instance, the palms tend to be held open, the hands raised, whereas in the Cheng Man-ch'ing style the hand is aligned with the forearm. The form presented later in this book is the Cheng Man-ch'ing Short Form (see pages 62–63) with a short variation.

The form is broken down into postures – a misnomer, since the term "posture" implies a static pose, yet the body is static for a few moments only at the beginning and the end of the form. Postures are short sequences of movements given a descriptive name. Some names have evolved from imitations of the movements of birds or animals – Golden Rooster Stands On One Leg is a good example – while others, such as Push and Punch, describe what happens in the movement.

In tai chi the mind contributes as much as the muscles to every movement. Awareness is the force that

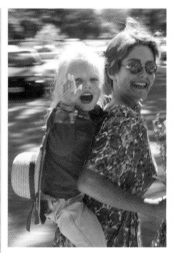

ABOVE *Maintaining harmony in movement is the basis of the graceful body movements of tai chi.*

directs energy to where it is needed and brings to life the spirit of each posture. It is mental awareness, rather than determination, that makes the largest contribution to training the body in balance and correcting the faults in posture that make a true alignment hard to achieve. Movement emerges from stillness, so fully understanding the need for correct alignment and posture when standing still are essential preparations for carrying out the movements of the form.

EARTH CENTER

The Earth holds you to its surface with a loving pull from its center. Through this idea tai chi encourages a healthy relationship with gravity. Cultivate this by imagining a connection from your feet to the center of the Earth's core, and by extending feeling downward from your feet. Visualize light beams joining you to the Earth's center.

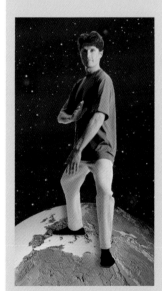

ABOVE *Encourage your sense of gravity by imagining a connection from your feet to the Earth's core.*

PREPARING FOR PRACTICE

In the form the attention needs to be in many places at once. Internally, a mental awareness is called upon to make an essential contribution to every movement. You need to feel a connection from your feet down to the center of the Earth, and its link to the pelvis, along the spine, and through the top of your head to an imaginary gateway to the cosmos which lies directly above it. Some of the time your focus also needs to be directed outward, for the floor on which you perform tai chi is a compass, providing external references for orientation.

Internal reference points

Moving or still, you are always connected to your center. Making the connection physical, by aligning your body from the top of your head to your feet on the earth center, gives you a sense of centralized equilibrium. Attune to this alignment mentally and it becomes something that is always with you. Then each step you take, each move you make, each direction you face comes from a sense of balance. Experiencing the world from this position is being at the center of your circle.

The higher extension point lies about 18 inches above the head, bordering the aura that surrounds the body. It links the cosmos to the body and indirectly to the Earth through the spine and pelvis. Directing your awareness to this point lifts your spirit through the top of your head.

The hands are sensors – they are human antennae. Always be aware of their primary function in tai chi movements, as givers and receivers.

The lower tantien energy center lies halfway between the top of the head and the feet. Also called the "sea of chi," it is the body's battery. Focusing attention here awakens its role as distrbutor of chi.

The top of the head is linked by the spine to the coccyx (tail bone), joining the spirit of the universe to the matter of the Earth. Feel it as soft and lifted from above. Directing awareness to it helps maintain a live, dynamic pathway along the spine.

The sacrum is the lower part of the spine that is built into the pelvis. In tai chi it connects the spine to the earth, symbolized by the legs and feet. Directing the awareness to the sacrum makes for effective grounding.

The feet are terminals through which the body becomes a conductor for power from the Earth. Imagine a gateway in each foot. All movements in tai chi come from the feet, which keep the body earthed and grounded. Directing the attention to the legs and feet encourages earthing.

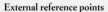

External reference points

The form starts as if the player stands in the center of a circle facing north. The other directions are external references to the choreography of the form. The tradition of facing north is said to derive from the idea of aligning with a cosmic center – the Pole Star, which appears as an anchor in the firmament and that navigators in the northern hemisphere use to find true north. It is not essential to begin the form facing north, but to follow the directions for the postures and movements on pages 62–115, it is necessary to choose a direction and call it north.

The Language of Tai Chi Movements

THERE ARE NO *unconsidered movements in tai chi. Every circling of an arm, every bending of a knee has its meaning, and as the body moves, it forms a succession of different shapes, each of which makes a statement. Tai chi uses body shape to express the mind's intentions, and remarkable small changes in shape can have a major emotional effect. Tai chi merges body and mind to create a language of body shapes which, performed in set sequences, tell a story.*

A STANDING MEDITATION

Every physical and mental movement in this standing meditation is found in the form. As it ends, direct your awareness to the higher extension point at the edge of your aura about 18 inches above your head. You are a unified organism, linked from the center of the Earth to the sky.

1 *Stand comfortably with your feet about one shoulder width apart. Slowly rock onto the balls of your feet, then move your weight back to the heels. Repeat several times, finishing with a sense of even weight distribution.*

2 *Bring your awareness to your sacrum (at the base of the spine), perhaps resting the back of your hand there. Feel the triangle made by your right foot, your left foot and your sacrum, and imagine it as your base.*

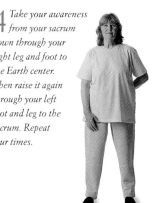

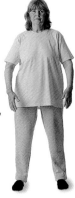

3 *Imagine gateways into the Earth passing through your feet. Through them your consciousness can move into the Earth, and the Earth into you.*

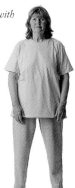

4 *Take your awareness from your sacrum down through your right leg and foot to the Earth center. Then raise it again through your left foot and leg to the sacrum. Repeat four times.*

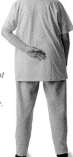

5 *Soften (focus on relaxing) the top of your head. Feel its link with the sacrum and the connection between sacrum, feet, and Earth. Feel a connection from the Earth center to the top of your head.*

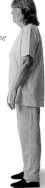

6 *Imagine your arms are rooted in your spine and that they branch out, opening at the shoulder, elbow, and wrist joints, and into the hands.*

7 *Make a space between each finger and relax the soft flesh around the hard bones of your hands, feeling the contrast.*

8 *Point your hands toward the ground and imagine your fingers having roots that extend into the Earth.*

BODY SHAPE – BODY MESSAGE

In the form different expressions are conveyed through palms, fingers, and fists. In White Crane Spreads Wings on page 74, one hand turns up to the sky as a conductor for cosmic energy, and the other faces the Earth to conduct Earth energy. In Push on page 69 energy travels from the Earth through the outward-facing palms. Discover the possibilities of expression through palms, fingers, and fist for yourself by exploring them as shown below; then put them into practice through the hand-position exercises Familiarize yourself with the way different hand shapes make you feel, exploring your own ideas. Then try different foot positions.

SOFTENING

"To soften" is a tai chi term meaning to focus on relaxing mentally and physically.

Softening the top of the head

A thin sheet of muscle covers the back of the head and most of the forehead. Contracting and relaxing softens the top of the head and stimulates blood flow to the scalp and head. Softening the crown forges the essential link between body and spirit, Earth, and cosmos.

Softening the hips

Imagine your hips are as pliable as a child's. To soften them is to relax every muscle, and to dissolve internal resistance to opening them, widening their range of movements.

FINGERS AND FIST

Fingers
Lift one arm to shoulder height and look along it toward the horizon with your fingers extended. Point each finger in turn at the horizon. Consider how each finger feels. Repeat with the other arm.

Fist
Make a fist with one hand. It should be soft and comfortable, with the thumb tucked outside the knuckles. Play with it, thinking about how it feels to you. Then repeat with the other hand.

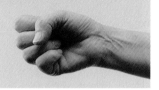

PALMS

1. Lift your arms in front of you and turn your palms toward you. Try to sense containment and holding in this position, called "palms facing." Now turn the palms toward the ground and notice the difference in feeling. Repeat the two palm positions.

2. Rotate your palms to face outward. This position carries a sense of energy moving out (try waving to someone with your palm facing).

3. Rest your arms by your sides briefly.

HAND POSITIONS

1. Stand comfortably and think of your internal reference points (see page 45). Turn both palms toward you and try to feel what this shape gives you.

2. Turn one palm up as if in dialog with the sky, and turn the other to face out – a position called "palm away" – as if communicating with the surrounding space. Feel what this gives you.

3. Drop the hand turned palm away and roll it to face palm down as if in dialog with the earth. Bring the palm you turned skyward to face your chest. Notice the feelings produced by the new hand shapes.

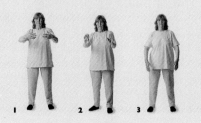

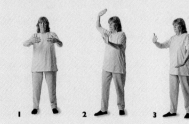

Eight Basic Postures

CENTURIES BEFORE MODERN *tai chi forms evolved, the writers of the classic texts spoke
of the "Thirteen Patterns" of tai chi. These patterns were sequences of movements making
up eight fundamental postures and five basic steps. The Thirteen Patterns are as relevant today
as they were when they were first worked out hundreds of years ago, for a sure way to develop
confidence and expertise in tai chi is by devoting plenty of time and practice to the basic
footwork and hand movements.*

THE FOUR PRIMARY POSTURES

1 Ward off (peng)

TRIGRAM: *Ch'ien, heaven, or spaciousness*

ATTRIBUTE: *Strong*

Ward Off energy is sometimes likened to water supporting a boat. It is something that fills the entire body from the inside. It imparts a feeling of buoyant, natural strength and creates space. Variations on this primary posture, Ward Off Left and Ward Off Right, appear at the beginning of the Short Form (see pages 66–67), where they fill the body with bouncy, springlike energy.

2 Rollback (lu)

TRIGRAM: *K'un, receptivity, Earth*

ATTRIBUTE: *Yielding*

Rollback is a protector that delivers a sense of choice. It actively invites incoming energy to the point where it exhausts itself. In neutralizing the incoming energy, it creates a place of choice from where a counter movement or a letting go offer equal possibilities. The second primary movement after Ward Off Left, it follows Ward Off Right on page 68, and is repeated four more times.

3 Press (chi)

TRIGRAM: *K'an, water*

ATTRIBUTE: *Flowing penetration*

Press is like a combination of Ward Off and Push: one arm wards off while the other pushes. It displays a bursting forward of energy up, down, or along, yet it retains a contained shape with which an incoming force may be met and repelled. It follows Rollback on page 68, and is repeated four times in the form. It enhances the bouncy, springlike energy of Ward Off and develops a reactive force.

4 Push (an)

TRIGRAM: *Li, fire, or vitality*

ATTRIBUTE: *Light-giving*

Push is a posture that sends energy outward. The fire of the Earth is pulled up through the body by Push, and moved out through the hands, surrounding and consuming the space into which it moves. It is the fourth primary posture, appearing four times in the form, three times following Ward Off, Rollback, and Press (see pages 66–69). This ancient pattern of the four primary postures is collectively called Grasp Sparrow's Tail.

THE FOUR SECONDARY POSTURES

5 Pull (tsai)

TRIGRAM: *Sun, wind*

ATTRIBUTE: *Sensitivity*

Pull tips the balance. Joining with the momentum of something, it adds just enough of its own energy to topple or upset the balance. The first of the secondary postures, it occurs in Single Whip on page 70, when both hands pull to the diagonal; again at the end of the form in the first step of Bend Bow to Shoot Tiger on page 112, when the hands sweep down, pulling something to the earth.

6 Shoulder (kao)

TRIGRAM: *Ken, mountain*

ATTRIBUTE: *Stillness and stability*

Shoulder stroke is a dynamic expression of solid Earth strength, using the weight and momentum of the whole body through the shoulder and upper back. The last of the secondary postures, it appears on page 73, where it makes you aware of your own physical strength.

7 Split (lieh)

TRIGRAM: *Chen, thunder*

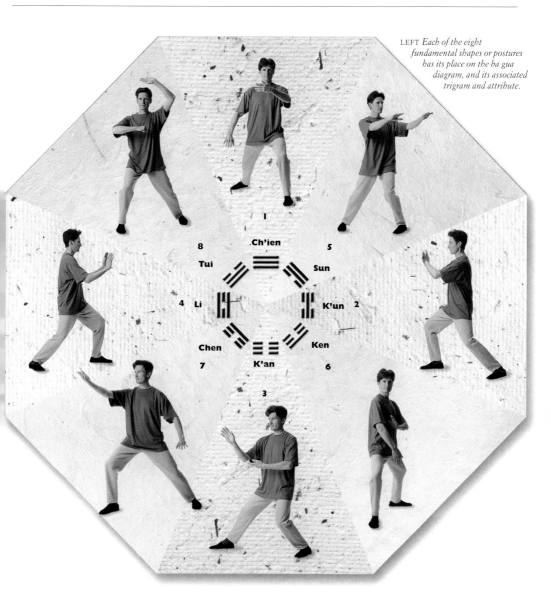

LEFT *Each of the eight fundamental shapes or postures has its place on the ba gua diagram, and its associated trigram and attribute.*

1

8 Ch'ien 5

Tui Sun

4 Li K'un 2

Chen Ken

7 K'an 6

3

ATTRIBUTE: *Arousing energy*

The secondary posture Split is the explosive force that moves in opposite directions from the same central, spinning source. It appears most spectacularly in the form in Diagonal Flying on pages 86–87.

8 Elbow (tsou)

TRIGRAM: *Tui, lake*

ATTRIBUTE: *Joy*

Short, sharp, and decisive, Elbow Stroke makes use of the energy generated as the arm folds at the elbow. The elbow is presented projecting forward from the body. As it unfolds, the fist is released to chop up or downward, and its movements can alternate with those of the elbow. Elbow appears in the second part of Turn Body, Chop, and Push on page 97.

49

The Stances

IN TAI CHI *the Earth is seen as a living organism with its own life force or chi, so that maintaining a strong connection between the body and the Earth is essential to health. An important aim of tai chi practice is to establish channels into the Earth through which good nourishment can be obtained from the mother lode of life energy. The legs and feet, therefore, have a fundamental role in tai chi, and to work on their connection to the Earth is to shape the fundamental building blocks of the art. Central to this process is the concept of grounding, or earthing.*

In tai chi, rooting is a physical process that encourages a condition of grounding. A well-based person gives the impression of having a relaxed solidity, of being in touch with the naturally strong part of the self. Being firmly grounded means that the body becomes the meeting place between the solid spirit of the Earth and the cosmic spirit of the heavens.

Practice begins with techniques aimed at creating central equilibrium (see page 52) and establishing a link with the Earth center. The stances and movements on the next pages are physical expressions of Earthing. Tai chi movements can feel awkward at first, but they encourage grounding and beginners soon feel more balanced and earthed. The mind benefits, as grounding encourages honesty and realism, and the dynamic ability to meet challenges.

THE BASIC STANCES

A movement must be based on the correct stance or foot position. The five basic stances are illustrated here. Practice each of these stances many times, moving the weight from side to side and front to back while keeping the feet still, in order to get used to how the stances feel. When these foot positions occur during the form (see pages 62–115), instructions are given for movements of weight and balance.

1 Parallel stance
Stand with the feet one shoulder's width apart and parallel (heels and toes aligned). This stance is found in the Beginning posture on pages 64–65, and in Crossing Hands on pages 81 and 114.

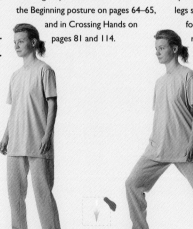

2 Bow and arrow (mountain-climbing) stance
Stand with your feet one shoulder width apart and parallel (toes and heels aligned), legs slightly bent at the knees. Turn your left foot out to a 45° angle, then lift your right foot and place it two shoulder widths in front of it. Bend your front knee and almost straighten your back (left leg) to give forward momentum like an arrow. Your waist and hips face the direction of your front (right) leg. Repeat the stance, stepping forward with your left leg. This stance occurs often in the form, notably in the four primary postures: Ward Off, Rollback, Press, and Push, which are repeated in the form.

THE BASIC STANCES

3 The cat stance

In this stance the feet make an L-shape. Stand, with the feet together, and turn the left foot out at a 90° angle. Move most of your weight onto your left leg. Lift your right foot, take a step forward and lift the heel so that just the ball of the foot touches the ground, and align your hips at a 45° angle to your right foot. Now repeat the posture, moving your weight onto your right leg, lifting your left heel, and aligning your hips at a 45° angle to your left foot. The cat stance appears in step 3 of White Crane Spreads Wings on page 74.

4 The heel stance

The feet make an L-shape in this stance, forming a 90° angle to each other, but the toes are lifted. Stand feet together and move most of your weight onto your left leg. Lifting the toes of your right foot, pivot on the heel until your feet form a 90° angle (making an L-shape). Keeping just the heel of your right (front) foot touching the floor, align your hips at an angle of 45° to it. Hold the posture, then repeat it, moving your weight onto your right leg and lifting your left toes. The heel stance appears in step 2 of Lifting Hands on page 72.

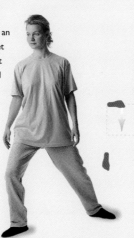

5 The T-stance

Despite its name, the feet form an L-shape in this stance. Stand feet together and turn your left foot out at a 90° angle. Step forward with your right foot and place it two shoulder widths in front of your left foot. Move 70% of your weight onto your right leg, then align your pelvis at an angle of 45° to your front foot. The T-stance appears in step 3 of Shoulder Stroke on page 73.

BUBBLING WELL

The connection between the body and the Earth center, described on pages 44–5, is traditionally held to take place through the point on the foot called the Yongquan, meaning "Bubbling Well." The Yongquan is a gateway in each foot through which you direct your awareness into the Earth, and where Earth energy can bubble up into your body.

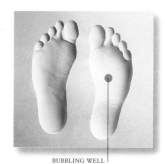

BUBBLING WELL

Stepping

IT MAY SEEM *strange to have to learn to walk again before starting the form, but mastering the principles of stepping is the key to performing the postures successfully. In tai chi the whole person, mind and body, takes part in every step. Here, the complex art of stepping is analyzed, and exercises help newcomers to tai chi to move with poise and grace. Learning to turn a stride or a bouncy step into a slow, steady glide is like practicing scales when learning music. It takes persistent hard work, which is clearly worthwhile when it comes to playing the piece.*

FIVE BASIC STEPS

Central equilibrium (see page 14) is a constant in all stepping, with its presence clearly marked at every moment. Before you move, picture a dividing line between the left and right sides of your body: as you move, you gain central equilibrium on one side, freeing the other to step.

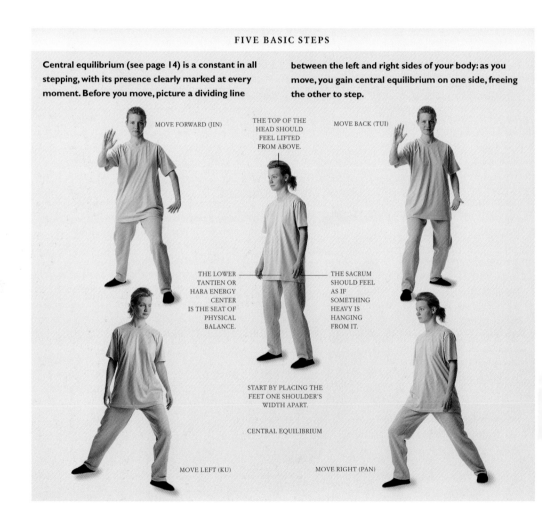

MOVE FORWARD (JIN)

THE TOP OF THE HEAD SHOULD FEEL LIFTED FROM ABOVE.

MOVE BACK (TUI)

THE LOWER TANTIEN OR HARA ENERGY CENTER IS THE SEAT OF PHYSICAL BALANCE.

THE SACRUM SHOULD FEEL AS IF SOMETHING HEAVY IS HANGING FROM IT.

START BY PLACING THE FEET ONE SHOULDER'S WIDTH APART.

CENTRAL EQUILIBRIUM

MOVE LEFT (KU)

MOVE RIGHT (PAN)

A PRACTICED STEP

The aspects of tai chi covered on the preceding pages, such as posture, central alignment, and stance, all contribute to the ability to step correctly. In tai chi, a step is far from the mechanical lifting and replacing of a foot as most people understand the term, but a steady, rhythmic progression of the weight from front to back and left to right. When performed by a practiced artist the legs may be seen to move, but the whole body from the feet to the crown of the head appears to stay in one plane, in line with the ground, and does not bob up and down. So although stepping backward, forward, and to either side may seem second nature, in tai chi these complex movements need thought and practice.

STEPPING WITH THE BOW AND ARROW STANCE

This stance occurs most often in the form, and involves transferring weight from side to side and front to back while moving the legs. To get a good feel for it, work at gliding the right foot forward while sitting into the left leg, and vice versa. Step 5 is the end of the stance. When you feel confident, go on to step 6, then practice it many times.

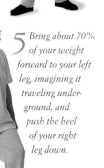

3 Turn your hips in the direction of the right foot, turn the spine, and spiral your weight into that foot. Lift your left heel.

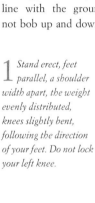

1 Stand erect, feet parallel, a shoulder width apart, the weight evenly distributed, knees slightly bent, following the direction of your feet. Do not lock your left knee.

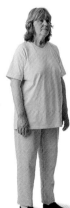

2 Sit into your left leg and turn your right foot 90° to the right, pivoting on the heel.

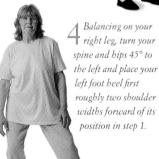

4 Balancing on your right leg, turn your spine and hips 45° to the left and place your left foot heel first roughly two shoulder widths forward of its position in step 1.

5 Bring about 70% of your weight forward to your left leg, imagining it traveling underground, and push the heel of your right leg down.

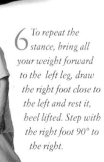

6 To repeat the stance, bring all your weight forward to the left leg, draw the right foot close to the left and rest it, heel lifted. Step with the right foot 90° to the right.

Balanced Walking

THE EXERCISES IN *balanced walking on these pages put the principles of tai chi stepping into practice. In the form, however, the weight and balance must also be moved while taking steps in all directions. This can be mastered only by learning a number of movements.*

When you feel confident about stepping, practice walking in a balanced way forward, then backward; then take several steps to the left and to the right. Take steps of a manageable size, and move slowly and smoothly, making sure of the ground before stepping. When you feel you can perform a balanced walk in each direction, experiment with stepping in any combination you like.

Forward

1 *Stand erect and correctly aligned. Sit into your right leg so you can release the left leg to step.*

2 *Drop your spine and step forward with your left leg. Place the heel first, then the whole foot. Keep your weight on the back leg as you step.*

3 *Check your balance by releasing the front foot, then putting it down, as if testing the ground.*

FORWARD

If you resist the impulse to lift your body as you step, you will notice the muscles in your legs working to move your leg forward and you will not bob up between steps. Your feet do not have to be parallel when you step forward or to the side. Take small steps at first.

4 *Keeping both legs still, transfer your weight to your left leg. Imagine it moving underground. Feel the right leg being released, ready to step.*

5 *Step forward, keeping your trunk in the same low position.*

6 *Continue to step with balance, never letting your body weight fall on the leading foot. Notice how you drop lower to take longer steps.*

BACKWARD

Plant your weight and balance in one leg and imagine testing the ground before committing weight to it. Stepping back with the feet parallel helps you move faster and more easily. This technique exercises the ankle joints, and opens the spine.

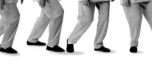

Backward

1 *Sit deeply into your right leg and take a small step backward with the left foot, toes touching the ground first. If you step too far back, you will not be able to rest the foot flat on the ground.*

2 *Check your balance by releasing the back foot, then putting it down as if testing the ground.*

3 *Carefully move your weight from front leg to back, imagining it traveling underground. Step back with the right foot, placing the toes down first.*

4 *Continue to step, keeping your center of gravity low so you do not bob up between steps. Then try stepping backward with your feet parallel.*

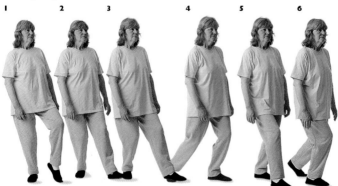

THE VOCABULARY OF MOVEMENT

Over the centuries, names have been given to tai chi's special movements. "Sitting" the weight into a leg and "folding in" the hips are two earthing movements which may need practice. Rather than view the legs as something you balance on, like stilts, you need to feel their dynamic relationship with the Earth. The body's weight and the mind's awareness may be visualized as a liquid pouring into the Earth; and the legs as channels conducting Earth energy up into the body through a gateway in the feet.

Sitting into a leg

Many postures instruct you to "sit into" the left or right leg. With your feet firmly planted, drop your spine earthward while bending the knees. This puts you in a semi-sitting position. Focus on the relationship between the sacrum, the feet, and the Earth. They make a strong foundation, like the base of a pyramid through which you feel grounded, yet lifted through the spine and the head. When you feel comfortable sitting into both legs, practice sitting into the left leg, then the right.

Folding in the hips

This movement earths the legs and feet, while granting mobility to the part of the body above the pelvis. Plant your feet firmly on the floor, imagine your hip joints have softened, drop your spine, bend your knees, and begin to squat. Incline your spine slightly forward, until there is just a finger-width of space between your lower pelvis and your upper thigh.

Hips

To open a joint is to remind it of its freedom to move. In order to open the hips, stand erect with your feet a shoulder's width apart and your knees slightly bent, and tuck your pelvis inward slightly. Breathe normally, emphasizing the out-breath and focus on relaxing all the muscles in your hips, abdomen, pelvis, and upper thighs. This allows the joints easy, unrestricted movement.

Palms

This is a fluid movement and it depends on the wrist being softened. To do this, hold your arms out in front of your body and focus your awareness on dispelling tension in muscles, tendons, and bones. Imagine energy flowing into and out of the secondary heart energy center in your palms. When your wrists are fully relaxed, you find your hands move smoothly up and back, opening the palms outward.

Opening and closing

Open and closed are two of the seven basic qualities of tai chi (see pages 14–15), so some part of the body is always opening and closing during tai chi movements.

Sideways

1 *Sit into your right leg and take a small step to the left. The inside edge of the foot touches the ground first.*

2 *With all your weight on your front (right) leg, test your balance by releasing the left foot, then putting it down again.*

3 *Move your weight from right leg to left, imagining it traveling underground, then step right. Continue to step slowly, keeping your center of gravity low so you do not bob up between steps.*

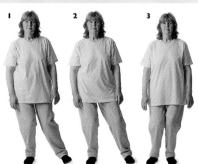

Key Moves

THESE TWO PAGES *present postures in which the legs and feet, once positioned, remain fixed while other parts of the body move. Practiced as solo postures, they offer an understanding of how the tai chi shapes work. Repeating these movements also generates energy, improves circulation, and warms the body. The first three exercises are characterized by repeated turning of the spine, and the different hand shapes express the energy generated by the moving spine. In Push, however, the body remains facing forward while moving forward and back.*

Begin each exercise by standing with the feet one shoulder width apart; turn the left foot out to a 45° angle, then move into a bow and arrow stance with the right leg two shoulder widths forward, toes facing ahead, and transfer 70% of your weight to it. (The front foot, pointing in any direction, is the base line, and all other directions are given in relation to it.)

ROLLBACK

For all moves keep a sense of soft fluidity, like waves rolling back and forth on the shore.

Right side (not pictured)

1 *With hips and pelvis as a guide, turn your spine toward the front right diagonal. The right arm, palm up, extends along the diagonal, and the left hand rests palm down opposite the middle of the body and the right elbow.*

2 *Keeping your weight mainly forward in your right leg, turn to face the front and roll your right palm to face down and the left palm to face up.*

3 *Continue turning left and back by bringing 70% into your back, left leg. The left arm unfolds from the elbow and the right arm folds in at the elbow.*

4 *Roll the right palm up and left palm down as you return 70% of your weight to the front (right) leg and once again turn to the front right diagonal as in step 1.*

Left side (pictured below)

1 *This time, with left leg forward, turn your spine left, extending your left arm, palm up along the front diagonal and rest the right hand, palm down, opposite the middle of the body and the left elbow.*

2 *Keeping your weight mainly forward, in your left leg, turn to face the front and roll your left palm to face down and right palm to face up.*

3 *Continue turning right and back, by bringing 70% of your weight into your back, right, leg. The right arm unfolds from the elbow while the left arm folds in at the elbow. Roll the left palm up and right palm down as you return 70% of your weight to the front (left) leg and once again turn to the front left diagonal.*

1

2

3

PRESS AND ROLLBACK

Press first appears on page 69 and occurs four times in the form, always following Rollback. In this exercise the hands join at the palms to press-forward, directing energy outward. The movements combine Press and Rollback in one continuous exercise, so that at the end of step 2 you release the press and follow with step 1 of Rollback. Repeat this pattern (rollback, press, rollback, press) continuously on the left and then the right for as long as you like.

PUSH

In this exercise the body remains facing forward. The push occurs in step 3 when the back leg pushes the body forward. After step 3, return to step 1 and repeat the movement over and over, generating a flowing, wavelike motion. Push appears four times in the form, first on page 69.

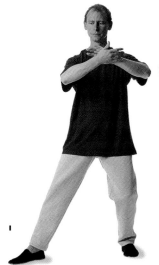

Right side

1 *Repeat steps 1 and 2 of Rollback, then bring the left hand to meet the right with the heels of the palms joining as you begin moving your weight forward to your right leg and turn to the right as far as your hips comfortably allow.*

2 *Press well forward during this movement. When 70% of your weight is forward, release your hands from their press position and extend the right arm, palm facing up, along the front right diagonal, and rest the left hand palm down opposite the middle of the body, as in step 1 of Rollback.*

Left side

Pause after performing the exercise on one side, rub your legs, then start again with the left foot forward.

1–3 *Repeat steps 1 and 2 of Rollback, then bring your right hand to meet the left, joining the heels of the palms as you begin to move your weight forward to the left leg and turn to the left as far as you can.*

4 *When 70% of your weight is on your front (left) leg, release your hands and extend your left arm, palm up, along the front left diagonal, resting the right hand palm down opposite the middle of the body and the left elbow. From here, follow with step 2 of the Rollback mirror image. Continue repeating steps 1–4 for as long as you wish.*

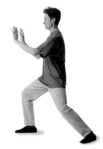

1 *Drop your elbows and lift both arms so that our hands are raised with the palms opposite your shoulders and facing outward.*

2 *Sit 70% of your weight on your back (left) leg and imagine it passing through your left foot into the earth. Keep the front right leg bent at the knee. At the same time, soften (relax) your shoulders, and, elbows leading, bring your hands toward your body in a downward-curving arc.*

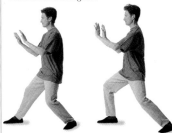

3 *Ease your weight forward to your front leg by straightening your back leg, while imagining the weight traveling underground. Lift your hands up to the front and rest them, palms facing outward, opposite your shoulders as in step 1.*

57

Warm-Up Movements

THE FOLLOWING FOUR *pages illustrate and give step-by-step instructions for 12 sets*
of movements that make an excellent warm-up sequence before beginning the form.
They exercise the body from head to toe, rotating the spine, stretching muscles and joints,
and stimulating the nervous system and the circulation of blood, tissue fluid, and life energy.
They also make a helpful preparation for the Short Form sequence (pages 62–115).

TURNING

This turn exercises the spine and
massages the kidneys, and relaxes
the body as a whole.

Stand comfortably upright with feet
parallel and one shoulder width apart.
Rotate the spine, first left and then right.
Let the arms swing with the turn and let
the weight shift from one leg to the other.

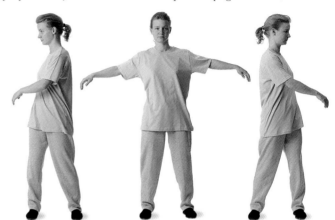

THE RAINBOW CIRCLE

This exercise stretches the spine and
the legs, and massages the liver.

1 Lift both arms, palms facing forward,
and keeping them parallel, paint an
imaginary rainbow with them from
horizon to horizon. As they fall to the
left, bend your spine left and, keeping

your legs straight, drop from the hips and
continue sweeping your arms as if painting
the bottom half of a circular rainbow.

2 When you have painted three to five
circles from left to right, interrupt the
movement on the downward sweep and
rest with your body dropped forward and
your arms touching the bottom of the arc,
to relax your face, neck, and shoulders.
Then swing round and up, painting the
circle from right to left.

3 Finish by resting briefly in the
forward bend position, then drop
right down into a squat, lifting your
hands at the same time as if you were
lifting a weight. Finally, raise your legs
and stand for a while with your knees
slightly bent and your palms facing your
abdomen at the level of the lower tantien.

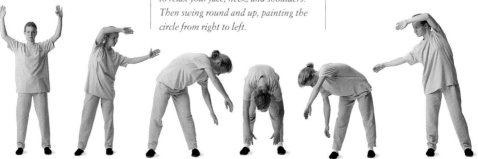

WILD HORSE

These rotations mobilize the hip joints and develop balance. When practicing, do not be alarmed by the sound of the hip joints moving in their sockets.

1 *Seating your balance in your left leg, rotate your right leg, moving it like a horse pawing the ground, although, while circling, your foot must not touch the ground. Repeat the exercise, circling the leg in the opposite direction.*

2 *Repeat step 1 with your balance in your right leg and rotating your left leg.*

3 *Lift your right leg, bending the knee. Relaxing the lower leg and*

foot, rotate the hip joint by describing an elliptical shape with the knee, three times clockwise and three times counterclockwise, then rest.

4 *Transfer your balance to your right leg and repeat step 3 with the left leg.*

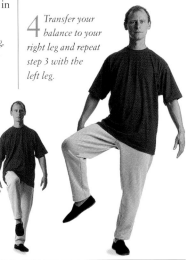

SAWING WOOD

This exercise encourages grounding and introduces you to the characteristic use of legs, hips, and feet.

Adopt a bow and arrow stance with your right leg forward. Swiftly move your weight forward to the right leg and back to the left leg, as if you were cutting across a tree trunk with a large, two-person saw. Swing your arms with the rhythm generated by the movement of weight from leg to leg. Keep your hips relaxed and your feet flat, with both knees slightly bent. Sit your body into the stance so your head and trunk do not bob up and down as your weight moves.

LEG SWINGS

These swings improve the balance, stretch the legs, develop mobility in the hips, and open the pelvis.

1 *Seat your weight in your left leg, and swing your right leg backward and forward, letting momentum build. As the foot comes forward, point the toes forward, and next time point the heel forward. After several swings, transfer your weight to your right leg and swing your left leg.*

2 *With your feet parallel and your weight seated in your left leg, lift your right leg and swing it out to the right side. Repeat three times. Approach the movement gently, achieving a comfortable swing, and you will feel the movement encouraging your hips and pelvis to open. Transfer your weight and balance to your right leg, and repeat the exercise swinging your left leg.*

CATHERINE WHEEL

This exercise opens the shoulder joint and stimulates the circulation in the arms.

Adopt a bow and arrow stance with your left leg forward. Rest your left hand on your left hip, make a loose fist with your right hand, and swing your right arm forward, up, back, and down, moving it like a Catherine wheel, building momentum. Continue for as long as you like, then repeat the exercise, swinging the arm back, up, forward, and down. Then step forward with your right leg, rest your right hand on your right hip, and repeat the whole exercise, swinging your left arm.

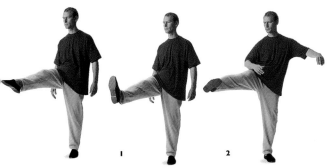

1   2

MERIDIAN ARM TWIST

This exercise revitalizes the arms and hands. It opens the meridians (channels of life energy) in the arms, and stretches the muscles, tendons, and ligaments.

1 Stand upright with your feet parallel and one shoulder's width apart. Drop the spine slightly and lift your arms up and out to shoulder height, palms facing down.

2 Turn your left palm up and look along your arm toward it. Relax the arm from the shoulder, imagining your fingers extending from your spine. The more you relax, the more you feel the stretch. At the same time, rotate your right arm along its length, first turning the palm down, then up and back as far as it can go. Hold for at least five seconds, then reverse the twist. Rotate your left palm down, up, and back, while turning to look down your right arm at your right hand, which is turned palm up. Look at each finger, feeling your consciousness extend to the tip.

3 Repeat step 2 three times finishing palms down as in step 1. Slowly raise your arms with the backs of the hands arcing toward each other until they nearly meet above your head.

4 Bring your hands down to touch the top of your head lightly. Keeping your feet flat, drop your spine as far as you can and push up with both hands, turning the palms up.

5 Let out a sigh, imagining that you are releasing unwanted, stuck, blocked, or gray life force, while releasing your arms and standing upright.

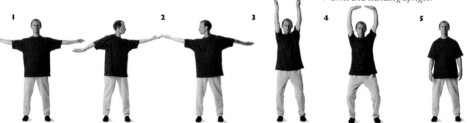

SPINE STRETCH PADDLE

This exercise opens and stretches the spine.

1 Stand comfortably upright, feet a shoulder's width apart. Interlock your fingers, and lift your arms just above your head, turning the joined palms upward. Drop your spine a little.

2 Focus your eyes on a point ahead and direct your attention to your neck. Move one elbow forward, down, back, and up, while moving the other back, up, down, and forward. This makes one stroke. Repeat three to five strokes on each side.

3 Drop your spine a little more, while raising your hands about 6 inches above your head. Direct your awareness to the middle of your spine, feeling a link between spine and hands. Paddle with your elbows, four strokes each side.

4 Drop your spine farther, push your hands to about 15 inches above your head, and keep your hips fixed facing the front. Direct your awareness to the sacrum, feeling a link moving up your spine, through your head to your hands. Paddle with your elbows, perhaps less vigorously.

5 Drop your spine as far as you can, push your hands as high as they will go. Feel the link from your coccyx (tail bone) to your hands. With a good sigh release your hands and rest.

6 Simply throw both arms up and out to the sides three or four times.

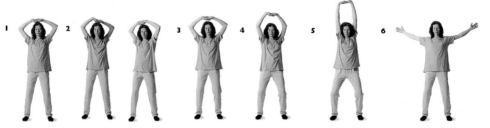

SPINAL WAVE

This exercise stimulates the thyroid gland, which has a role in the metabolism and digestion of sugars.

1 *Send your chin forward, and on an out-breath drop your head, drop your hips, and move your spine forward.*

2 *Tuck your chin in initially as you draw your breath in and move back to an upright position. This gives a wavelike motion up the spine. Repeat two more times.*

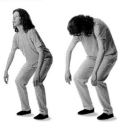

CLAPPING

This exercise encourages the chest to open and stale air to be expelled from the lungs. It stimulates the nerve endings and the circulation in the hands.

With the arms relaxed and comfortably extended, clap your hands together in front of your body to give a good slapping sound. Swing your arms back to clap behind the body, letting the breath out of your lungs. Repeat at least five times.

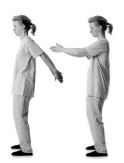

SNAKE SHAKE

This move improves the flexibility of the spine and massages the internal organs, refreshing them by increasing their supply of blood and tissue fluid. It is important to practice gently because the exercise massages the lungs vigorously.

1 *Stand comfortably upright and keep the rest of the body as still as possible while swinging the pelvis from side to side. Settle into this movement for a good minute.*

2 *From the sacrum at its base feel your whole spine begin to come to life in a rising wavelike motion as if a snake that lives in your pelvis winds its way all the way up to the top of your head.*

3 *The rising energy reaches the top of your head, softening the crown and pouring out like a soothing, cleansing*

liquid that washes over your body. Shake your body, keeping the feet flat on the ground and making the spine rise and fall energetically. Feel the shake through into your fingertips and keep it going for at least 30 seconds.

4 *Repeat steps 1–3 two more times, letting the shake continue for as long as you wish. Experiment with slow and quick shaking. Finish standing still, feeling your body working and the contrast between its still exterior and the movements of heart and lungs. Notice the vitality of your cells.*

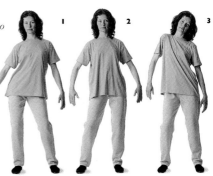

CLEARANCE

Release and clearance of stale energy is brought about by this vigorous arm movement.

Raise your right arm above your head. Bring it crashing down to stop abruptly opposite the pelvis, and accompany the move with a loud ssshhh as you expel air through your mouth. Raise your left arm above your head and repeat the movement. Repeat it five to ten times on each side. Imagine releasing any unwanted feelings and clearing your emotions.

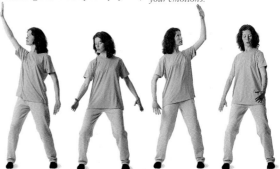

The Complete
Short Form

THE FORM – *the essence of tai chi – is the subject of the following pages. Each page illustrates, step by step, the sequence of postures that makes up one form. Guidelines are given to the mental awareness that, ideally, should accompany the postures. Tai chi is a holistic practice, which values both the mental and physical components; imagination and visualization make a great difference to the performance of the postures and their effectiveness in achieving health.*

The step-by-step instructions are written for individuals who want to practice alone at home or with friends in small groups. It is scarcely possible to learn tai chi without instruction from a teacher, but these pages can provide a useful framework for daily practice between sessions, for anyone unable to attend classes regularly, and those who have been learning tai chi for some time.

The form presented here is based on the Cheng Man-ch'ing style. A respected tai chi master who taught for many years in China, Cheng Man-ch'ing transformed the classic Yang tai chi style, shortening it and making it more concise. Anyone familiar with the Cheng Man-ch'ing Short Form will notice, however, that the sequence of movements and the positions of the hands presented in this book differ from the version they first learned.

In the late 1950s a disciple of Cheng Man-ch'ing, Dr. Chi Chiang-tao, introduced a new version of his teacher's form: he took a sequence of movements from the Yang Style Long Form and added it to Cheng Man-ch'ing's Short Form. Dr. Chi

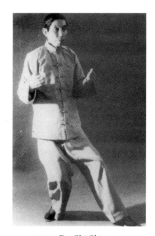

ABOVE *Dr. Chi Chiang-tao, author of the variation on Cheng Man-Ch'ing's short form illustrated in this book.*

decided to make this change for the benefit of his students' health. One posture he took from the Yang Style Long Form, called Needles at Sea Bottom, is especially beneficial for the internal organs, and the sequence improves both coordination and balance.

There are many ways of interpreting tai chi, and Chi Chiang-tao's variation of the Cheng Man-ch'ing Short Form is presented in a way that can be adapted to the needs of

individuals. Variations teach alternative ways of moving, and so broaden experience. A skillful teacher can assess students' needs and help them to discover the most appropriate techniques for them.

Although you can practice the tai chi form as a succession of purely physical movements, it also offers a spiritual dimension. The moments of stillness before the first posture and after the last, provide the player with a space in which to find an inner alignment of balance, mirrored by the standing posture. As the moves unfold, sensations of inner rhythms and cycles can reflect for the player a microcosmic "internal experience" that is part of a greater macrocosmic web of life.

Tai chi is not a religion and should not be practiced with the expectation of deep spiritual experiences, but opening oneself to the possibility of spiritual growth may prove to be rewarding. On one level, tai chi may provide a nonreligious antidote to the spiritually draining trends in modern living; and on another, it could blossom into a uniquely personal experience.

CHENG MAN-CH'ING'S ORIGINAL SEQUENCE

Illustrated here is the sequence of postures as found in the original Cheng Man-ch'ing form. Separate Left Foot on page 94 is followed by Turn and Kick With Heel, the first posture illustrated here. The sequence continues with Brush Left Knee and Push followed by Brush Right Knee and Push. The remainder of the form, from Brush Left Knee and Punch Downward on page 101 to Completion on page 115, follows Cheng Man-ch'ing's original sequence.

Turn and kick with heel

1 Balancing on your right leg, turn on the heel of your right foot so that it faces south, and kick with your heel toward the east.

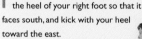

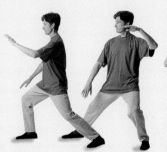

GUIDE TO THE SHORT FORM

• With daily practice it takes about one year to learn the Short Form.
• The complete Short Form sequence of postures takes 7–10 minutes to perform.
• Ideally, students should aim to practice once a day for perhaps 10 minutes at first, working up to perhaps a half hour a day or longer.
• The following pages give step-by-step guidelines for each movement in the sequence, but it is advisable to attend introductory courses and classes as well as practicing alone.
• The mental awareness guidelines are given as helpful support rather than as a definitive instruction.
• The Chi Chiang-tao variation begins with Brush Knee and Push (page 95) and ends with Brush Right Knee and Push (page 100).

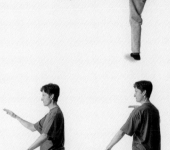

Brush left knee and push

2 Step forward into a bow and arrow stance, leading with your left leg, and push forward with your right hand as illustrated in Brush Left Knee and Push on pages 75 and 77.

Brush right knee and push

3 Turning your left foot to the left diagonal, facing southwest, bring your weight onto your left leg. Now release your right foot to step into a bow and arrow stance, brushing your right knee and pushing forward with your left hand.

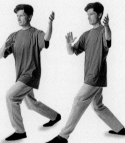

Beginning

IT IS IMPORTANT *from the very beginning of the form to work at developing awareness.
Begin this position by taking in the room, landscape, or cityscape in which one is practicing,
and thinking about the body's place in the space it occupies. Take as long as necessary to focus
fully on the present. The first step connects the body with the earth. It is followed by a
sequence of movements describing a cycle that draws up and in, then returns to the earth.
The movements are performed slowly and rhythmically in an unbroken flow.*

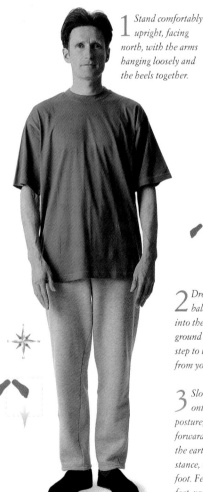

1 *Stand comfortably
upright, facing
north, with the arms
hanging loosely and
the heels together.*

BREATHING

From the beginning, become aware
of your breathing. Let your breath
enter your body and leave it
comfortably. Notice how your
breathing joins you to the space
around you. Take three successively
deeper, fuller breaths and relax a
little further with every out-breath.

2 *Drop your spine, as if seating all your
balance in your right leg and sending it
into the earth. Release your left foot from the
ground and, turning it to face directly north,
step to the left, resting it a shoulder width
from your right foot.*

3 *Slowly draw about 60% of your weight
onto your left leg, keeping it there through the
posture, and lift your arms by drawing your elbows
forward. Imagine yourself filling with energy from
the earth. Straighten your legs to a more upright
stance, moving your right foot parallel to your left
foot. Feel connected to the earth through your
feet, your hands, and the base of your spine.*

4 *Let your arms float upward, relax your wrists and the muscles of your arms, and imagine you are drawing energy from the earth up your spine and up through the space around you. Lift your arms until they are parallel to the ground, letting your hands droop.*

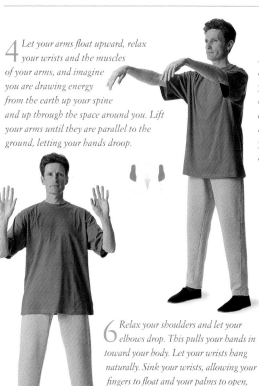

5 *Feel the connection from the earth through the center of your body to the crown of your head. It moves along your arms, and as it reaches your hands and fingers, let them float up until they are in line with your arms and parallel to the ground. Feel the Earth energy reach your fingertips.*

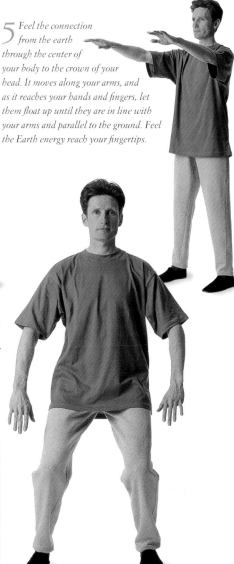

6 *Relax your shoulders and let your elbows drop. This pulls your hands in toward your body. Let your wrists hang naturally. Sink your wrists, allowing your fingers to float and your palms to open, facing forward. Pause to soften (relax) your whole being. Consider the miracle of your life, allowing feelings of joy to fill your body.*

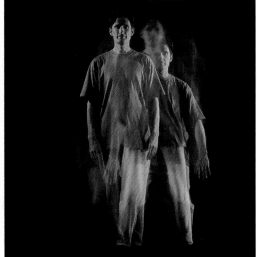

7 *Let your hands float down, to rest with your arms slightly lifted, your elbows slightly forward, completing the cycle and returning to earth. Let your spine drop as far as you comfortably can, so you finish almost sitting in a standing position. Your stance should be solid and your weight still distributed 60% on the left leg and 40% on the right. Spirit rising upward, feel youself earthed.*

Ward Off Left and Ward Off Right

START POSITION

WARD OFF LEFT *and Ward Off Right are variations on the primary posture Ward Off. Together with Rollback, Press, and Push (pages 68–69), these postures are collectively called Grasp Sparrow's Tail. They make up the four primary moves of the eight basic postures. Ward Off Left builds strength in the pelvis, seat of the hui yin and lower tantien energy centers, associated with sexual and creative energies. Ward Off Right is not just a mirror image of its predecessor; it takes the contained energy of Ward Off Left and develops it, giving a more outward expression of Ward Off, one of the primary moves.*

1 *From the semi-sitting position you held at the end of the first posture, with your weight distributed 60% on your left leg and 40% on your right, your arms lifted, and your elbows slightly forward, make a minor turn to the left.*

2 *Slowly move all your weight onto your left leg as you make a large turn 90° to the right, pivoting on your right heel and bringing the foot to rest facing east. Raise your right arm as if you were collecting a large ball beneath it, and support it by bringing your left arm beneath it.*

3 *Following the direction of your right foot, sit all your weight onto your right leg, allowing your left leg to rest behind with the heel lifted.*

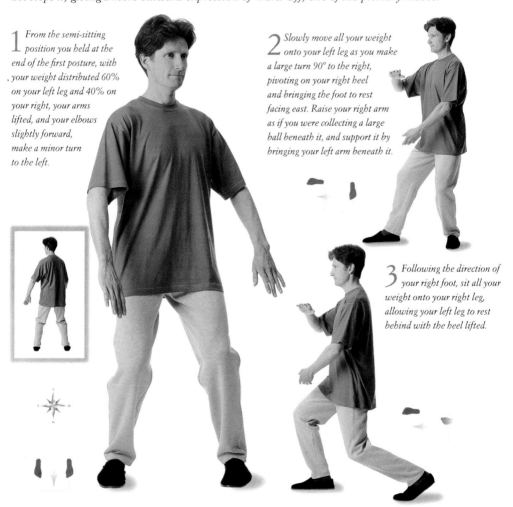

4 *Sitting into your right leg, release your left foot to step north into a bow and arrow stance, placing the heel down first. Your weight rests mainly on the back (right) leg. Your feet describe a 90° angle, a shoulder width apart and twice this distance front to back. Do not lock the front leg at the knee.*

WARD OFF RIGHT

START POSITION

Like a wave, these postures flow on from the end of the last. Begin by imagining oneself gathering the energy generated in Ward Off Left to mobilize it. Ward Off Right is the wave racing to the shore – it energizes the body by drawing up the creative sexual energy of Ward Off and giving it expression.

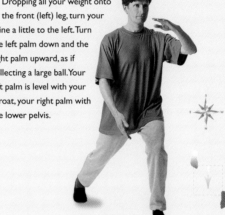

I Dropping all your weight onto the front (left) leg, turn your spine a little to the left. Turn the left palm down and the right palm upward, as if collecting a large ball. Your left palm is level with your throat, your right palm with the lower pelvis.

5 *Transfer your weight forward to your front leg, imagining it moving underground, while raising your left arm and lowering your right hand. Push down with your back foot, which straightens your back leg, turns your body to face north, and turns the toes of your back foot 45° to the northeast. Finish with your weight distributed 70% on the back (right) leg and 30% on the front leg.*

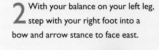

2 With your balance on your left leg, step with your right foot into a bow and arrow stance to face east.

3 Finish facing east, with 70% of your weight on the front (right) leg and 30% on the back leg. Your right arm leads up and away, your left arm following. This marks the end of the posture, which flows without a break into Rollback.

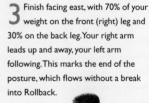

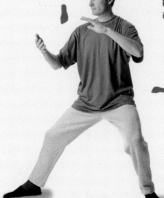

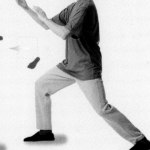

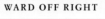

67

Rollback

THIS IS ONE *of the four primary postures. Rollback can receive or absorb a strike or push from an opponent, and offer a simultaneous counter. It teaches how to draw boundaries and hold one's space; and how to earth awkward incoming energy. As you begin, extend your awareness southeast along the diagonal. Let your mind travel with the spiraling, rolling movement, which gathers from the front right (southeast), carries back, and releases.*

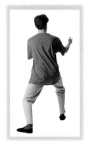

START POSITION

1 *While visualizing the wave breaking, remain anchored in the front (right) leg, relax, and make a small turn southeast, toward the diagonal running southeast–northwest. Your hands have dropped, the right hand into the position for shaking hands, and the left hand opposite the right elbow.*

2 *Simultaneously move your weight back along the diagonal, rotate your spine to the left, rotate your left forearm until the palm faces upward, and drop your right elbow to let the right hand float up. Finish with 70% of your weight on your back (left) leg, 30% on your front leg, your hips facing the northeast diagonal, the right palm facing north, and the fingers of your left hand near your right elbow.*

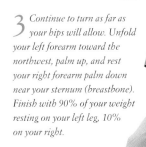

3 *Continue to turn as far as your hips will allow. Unfold your left forearm toward the northwest, palm up, and rest your right forearm palm down near your sternum (breastbone). Finish with 90% of your weight resting on your left leg, 10% on your right.*

VISUALIZATION

When you have become familiar with the whole posture, try to enhance its effects by visualizing a wave, which rises with Ward Off Right, breaks on the beach with the first part of Rollback, and washes back down the beach to the sea with the second part.

Press, Push

START POSITION

PRESS IS A *fabulous bursting forward of energy. All the cells of the body are energized, uniting to give a focused release of energy. Push, which follows Press, uses outgoing energy in a different way to produce a revitalizing effect on energy levels. It can be repeated as a solo exercise time and again, to improve focus and concentration and build life force. Physically, it is especially helpful in developing flexibility in the ankles.*

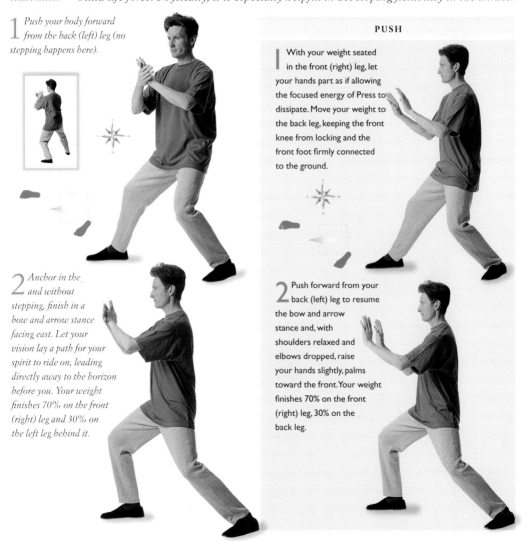

1 *Push your body forward from the back (left) leg (no stepping happens here).*

2 *Anchor in the and without stepping, finish in a bow and arrow stance facing east. Let your vision lay a path for your spirit to ride on, leading directly away to the horizon before you. Your weight finishes 70% on the front (right) leg and 30% on the left leg behind it.*

PUSH

I With your weight seated in the front (right) leg, let your hands part as if allowing the focused energy of Press to dissipate. Move your weight to the back leg, keeping the front knee from locking and the front foot firmly connected to the ground.

2 Push forward from your back (left) leg to resume the bow and arrow stance and, with shoulders relaxed and elbows dropped, raise your hands slightly, palms toward the front. Your weight finishes 70% on the front (right) leg, 30% on the back leg.

Single Whip

START POSITION

THIS FAMOUS POSTURE *occurs in all tai chi styles. It can be applied so that it contains each of the four secondary postures of the basic eight – pull, split, elbow, and shoulder – it could almost be said that knowing the form as far as this seventh posture is all that is necessary, as it embraces all the essential movements of tai chi. Single Whip develops focus, control, and balance, and encourages an opening and airing of the lungs.*

1 *Bring your balance solidly onto your left leg, which has the effect of extending your arms.*

2 *From your hips, turn your spine to the left, arms still reaching out as if throwing something to the northwest corner. Follow with your right foot, turning it through 90° so it finishes pointing toward north.*

3 *Your feet remain planted as your weight moves from left leg to right, and your spine rotates to the right as far as your hips allow. Fold in your right hip to allow spine and pelvis maximum turn.*

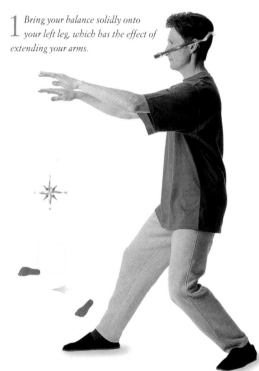

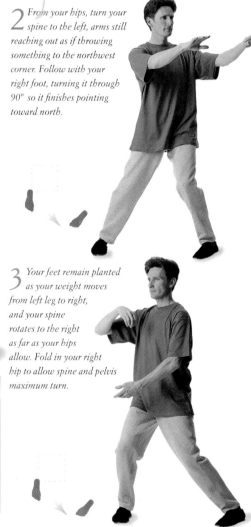

HANDS

Having cast the net during step 1, your hands catch hold of a ball as you turn right in step 3. As you finish turning, transform your right hand into a hook (right). During the left turn in step 4, the hands move in different directions.

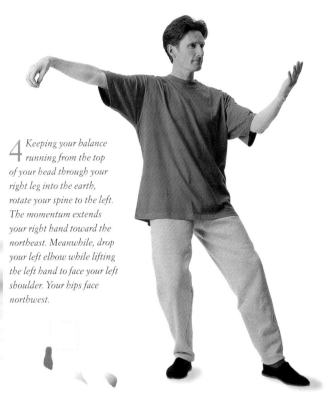

4 *Keeping your balance running from the top of your head through your right leg into the earth, rotate your spine to the left. The momentum extends your right hand toward the northeast. Meanwhile, drop your left elbow while lifting the left hand to face your left shoulder. Your hips face northwest.*

HANDS AND ARMS

During step 4 you make a hook (right) with your right hand. Feel how it becomes an anchor and a closed circuit, containing and recirculating energy to the left hand – which rises as your body turns, and leads. During step 5 your right arm remains out to the side, where it moved during step 4. Focus on how dark turns to light during this movement. As you straighten your right leg in step 6, your left hand turns from palm facing to palm away, and your awareness moves away as if you were gazing over a landscape. You may end step 6 by setting your wrist back to open the palm further.

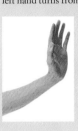

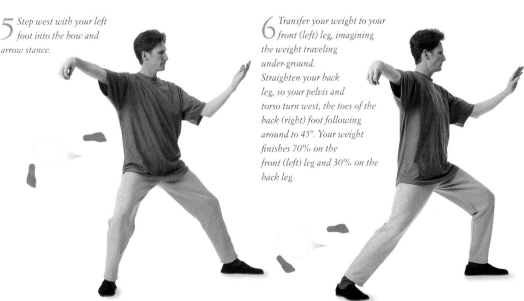

5 *Step west with your left foot into the bow and arrow stance.*

6 *Transfer your weight to your front (left) leg, imagining the weight traveling under-ground. Straighten your back leg, so your pelvis and torso turn west, the toes of the back (right) foot following around to 45°. Your weight finishes 70% on the front (left) leg and 30% on the back leg.*

71

Lifting Hands

THIS POSTURE DEVELOPS *the ability to open and close physically and mentally. It encourages deep relaxation and clarity of focus. During step 1, relax completely, allowing yourself to dissolve into the universe. Focus your awareness during step 2 on a point of star-like light about 18 inches from the fingertips of your right hand. Feel the contrast between this clear focus and the sensation of dispersion at the end of step 1.*

1 *Relaxing deeply onto your left leg, soften your arms, release your (right) hook hand, and begin turning your palms toward one another.*

Moving all your weight to your front leg, turn your hips to face northwest while moving your arms into an open gesture. Lift your right heel and pivot the foot.

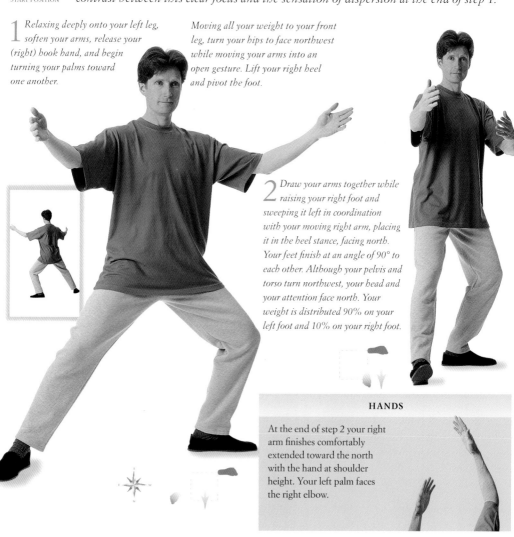

2 *Draw your arms together while raising your right foot and sweeping it left in coordination with your moving right arm, placing it in the heel stance, facing north. Your feet finish at an angle of 90° to each other. Although your pelvis and torso turn northwest, your head and your attention face north. Your weight is distributed 90% on your left foot and 10% on your right foot.*

HANDS

At the end of step 2 your right arm finishes comfortably extended toward the north with the hand at shoulder height. Your left palm faces the right elbow.

Shoulder Stroke

THIS IS ONE *of the secondary postures of the basic eight. It expresses solid, mobile power and helps people contact their own physical strength. As if pulling down from the point of light at the end of Lifting Hands, let your consciousness move through your left foot deep into the Earth's center. Focus on this sense of balance, directing your attention inward during step 1. You end step 2 in the T-stance. In step 3 you journey back from the center of the Earth.*

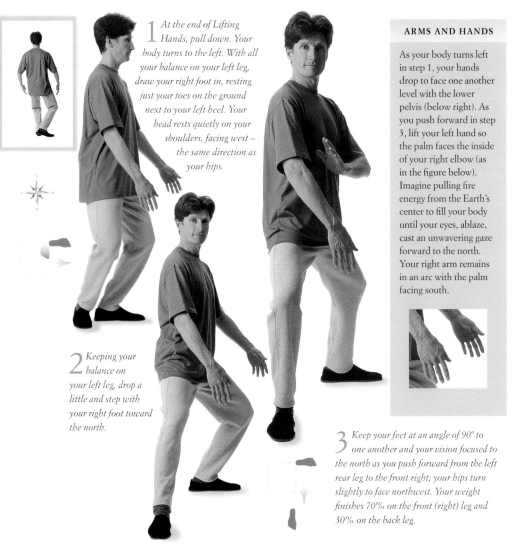

1 *At the end of Lifting Hands, pull down. Your body turns to the left. With all your balance on your left leg, draw your right foot in, resting just your toes on the ground next to your left heel. Your head rests quietly on your shoulders, facing west – the same direction as your hips.*

2 *Keeping your balance on your left leg, drop a little and step with your right foot toward the north.*

3 *Keep your feet at an angle of 90° to one another and your vision focused to the north as you push forward from the left rear leg to the front right; your hips turn slightly to face northwest. Your weight finishes 70% on the front (right) leg and 30% on the back leg.*

ARMS AND HANDS

As your body turns left in step 1, your hands drop to face one another level with the lower pelvis (below right). As you push forward in step 3, lift your left hand so the palm faces the inside of your right elbow (as in the figure below). Imagine pulling fire energy from the Earth's center to fill your body until your eyes, ablaze, cast an unwavering gaze forward to the north. Your right arm remains in an arc with the palm facing south.

White Crane Spreads Wings

THIS POSTURE INTRODUCES *a new stance – the cat stance. It encourages movement out into the world from a relaxed center. It also introduces a change in direction from north to west, and it is the first posture to actively open up the dimension of the sky, spreading the body between the earth and the heavens. This opens the front of the body, inviting the energy center at the solar plexus to shine.*

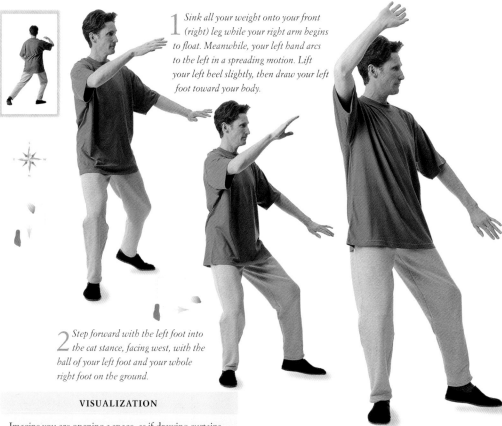

1 *Sink all your weight onto your front (right) leg while your right arm begins to float. Meanwhile, your left hand arcs to the left in a spreading motion. Lift your left heel slightly, then draw your left foot toward your body.*

2 *Step forward with the left foot into the cat stance, facing west, with the ball of your left foot and your whole right foot on the ground.*

VISUALIZATION

Imagine you are opening a space, as if drawing curtains apart, into which you carefully step and look. You might visualize a spiral of golden light running from your right hand, down your right arm, across your back, over your solar plexus and around your body, to finish by connecting into the lower left arm and hand.

3 *Your weight and balance stay on your back (right) leg. Your left foot is active, pushing to straighten the legs a little. As this is happening your left hand drops to the left, facing down and away from your body, while your right hand rotates upward, facing the sky. Your weight is distributed 90% on your right leg and 10% on your left.*

Brush Left Knee and Push

THE READY-FOR-ACTION *energy of White Crane Spreads Wings has a chance for expression in Brush Left Knee and Push, when something is caught and then sent. This posture develops coordination between left and right and encourages the qualities of receiving and giving.*

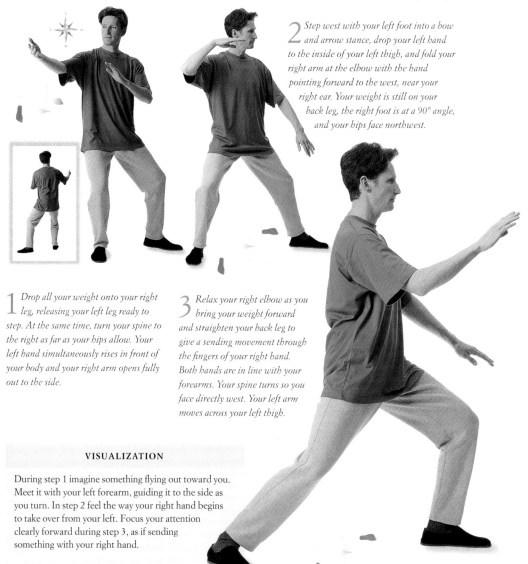

2 Step west with your left foot into a bow and arrow stance, drop your left hand to the inside of your left thigh, and fold your right arm at the elbow with the hand pointing forward to the west, near your right ear. Your weight is still on your back leg, the right foot is at a 90° angle, and your hips face northwest.

1 Drop all your weight onto your right leg, releasing your left leg ready to step. At the same time, turn your spine to the right as far as your hips allow. Your left hand simultaneously rises in front of your body and your right arm opens fully out to the side.

3 Relax your right elbow as you bring your weight forward and straighten your back leg to give a sending movement through the fingers of your right hand. Both hands are in line with your forearms. Your spine turns so you face directly west. Your left arm moves across your left thigh.

VISUALIZATION

During step 1 imagine something flying out toward you. Meet it with your left forearm, guiding it to the side as you turn. In step 2 feel the way your right hand begins to take over from your left. Focus your attention clearly forward during step 3, as if sending something with your right hand.

EALING TERTIARY COLLEGE
LEARNING RESOURCE CENTRE - EALING GREEN

Play Guitar

START POSITION

PLAY GUITAR ENCOURAGES *a light, open, balanced perspective. The posture is about stepping forward to catch something, so when making the first step, imagine reaching to touch something with the right hand. It trains coordination between stepping, momentum, and arm movement. Focus on timing, so that hands and heel all arrive in their final position together, like something clicking into place.*

1 *Sit into your front (left) leg and step up with your back (right) foot to rest it close to and slightly behind your left foot, at an angle of 45°.*

VISUALIZATION

Feel the contained space between your arms, and affirm your connection to the earth through your body. Imagine light pouring from your heart to fill the space created by your arms and hands. Let the light permeate your bones, blood, cells, and whole body, and feel it extend into the surrounding space.

2 *Transfer all your weight to your back (right) leg while extending your left arm so that the hand is at shoulder height and the elbow relaxed downward. Meanwhile, release your left foot to rest the heel a little forward and left of your right foot. Your right hand moves in and downward, resting opposite your left elbow. Finish with your hips facing northwest and 90% of your weight on your back (right) foot and 10% on your front foot.*

Brush Left Knee and Push (2)

THE VERSION OF *Brush Knee and Push on this page is similar to that on page 75, but it starts from a quieter place and makes use of the palms of the hands. Instead of catching something flying, as after White Crane Spreads Wings, imagine carrying back the light, open attitude of the last posture – the energy built up during Play Guitar is guided back by the left hand at the beginning of Brush Left Knee and sent out and forward by the right hand.*

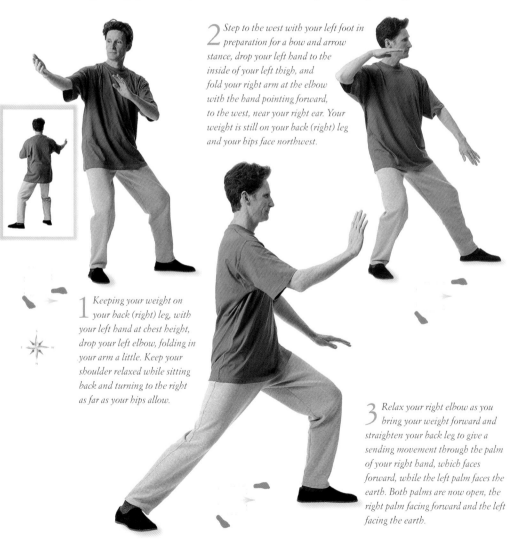

2 *Step to the west with your left foot in preparation for a bow and arrow stance, drop your left hand to the inside of your left thigh, and fold your right arm at the elbow with the hand pointing forward, to the west, near your right ear. Your weight is still on your back (right) leg and your hips face northwest.*

1 *Keeping your weight on your back (right) leg, with your left hand at chest height, drop your left elbow, folding in your arm a little. Keep your shoulder relaxed while sitting back and turning to the right as far as your hips allow.*

3 *Relax your right elbow as you bring your weight forward and straighten your back leg to give a sending movement through the palm of your right hand, which faces forward, while the left palm faces the earth. Both palms are now open, the right palm facing forward and the left facing the earth.*

Punch

THE FULL NAME *for this posture is Step Forward, Deflect Downward, Intercept, and Punch. Gathering root power, it moves into an earthy, heartfelt crescendo with the punch at the end. The use of the fist and the atmosphere of the final posture make a statement in the form. Punch is a gutsy posture, wonderful for coordination and balance, and it is a fine remedy for faintheartedness and a tentative approach to life. It embodies the soft, relaxation of yin energy with the outward going, harder yang force.*

1 *Bring most of your weight onto your back (right) leg, soften (relax) your left hand, and, making a fist of your right hand, move your right arm down to mirror the left. Pivoting on your left heel, turn your left foot to face the front left (southwest) diagonal, and rest it flat.*

2 *Follow the direction of your left foot with your pelvis and bring all your weight to sit into your left leg. Lift your right heel as your right leg rests behind.*

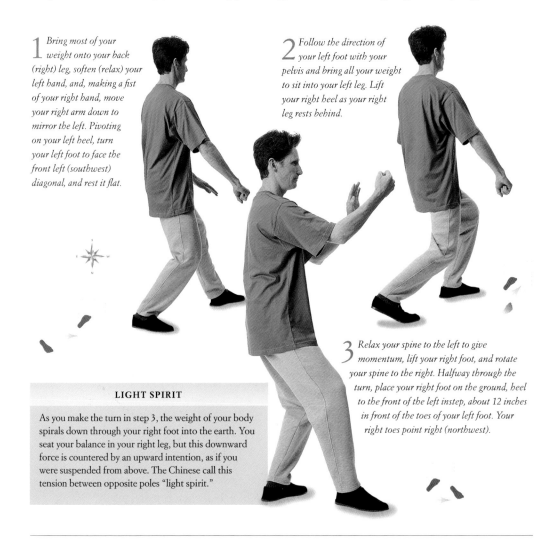

3 *Relax your spine to the left to give momentum, lift your right foot, and rotate your spine to the right. Halfway through the turn, place your right foot on the ground, heel to the front of the left instep, about 12 inches in front of the toes of your left foot. Your right toes point right (northwest).*

LIGHT SPIRIT

As you make the turn in step 3, the weight of your body spirals down through your right foot into the earth. You seat your balance in your right leg, but this downward force is countered by an upward intention, as if you were suspended from above. The Chinese call this tension between opposite poles "light spirit."

THE FIST IN TAI CHI

It is important to form the fist correctly. It should not be tense or tight, but soft, yet firm. The thumb bends at the joints, running across the outside of the last set of finger knuckles. The fingers must never curl around the thumb.

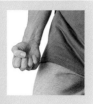

4 Turn your hips in the direction of your right foot, so your trunk faces northwest. Continue turning right and bring all your weight to your right foot, imagining it spiraling through your foot into the earth. Your left foot, heel raised, rests behind.

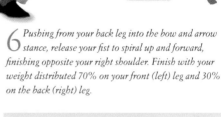

6 Pushing from your back leg into the bow and arrow stance, release your fist to spiral up and forward, finishing opposite your right shoulder. Finish with your weight distributed 70% on your front (left) leg and 30% on the back (right) leg.

5 Release your left foot to step forward and change your focus to the front (west), looking past your left hand.

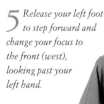

HANDS

From the beginning of the turn in step 3, sweep your right fist, hand upward, in an arc to drop down by your hip. Raise your left hand, so that as your hip drops, your left palm faces the right front diagonal. Follow this direction with your face and your eyes.

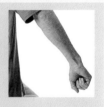

Your right hand, if you opened your fist, would face palm up. The root energy you gathered during step 1 is used in step 3 in painting the arc with your fist to link root (lower pelvis) to heart and back to root. Feel the stored power in your fist, and notice how your left hand emerges forward from the tail of this arc of power. Finish step 3 focusing toward the diagonal, eyes and left palm working together, and a clear alignment through your right side. Step 5 brings the left hand closer to the body. It finishes opposite your right elbow, and forward from the center of the chest.

Withdraw and Push

START POSITION

WITHDRAW AND PUSH *releases the energy of the punch at the end of the last posture in a beautiful gesture, then clears the space and fills it again, to give a new start. It teaches the mental and physical aspects of the qualities of full and empty. Feel the contrast between the fullness of the punch at the end of the last posture and the sense of release as you gently relax your fist hand in step 1.*

1 *Sitting into your left hip, turn a little to the left. Simultaneously release your fist, turning the palm of your right hand up slightly. Bring the left hand down, rotating the palm up, until the fingers lie just under your right elbow.*

2 *Bring the weight back onto your right leg and turning to the right, draw your right arm over your left hand as if clearing something from the forearm. Your hips now face north-west. Turn to the west and drop your left elbow so both arms are relaxed, with the palms at stomach height, turned up toward your face.*

3 *Relax your elbows, turn your palms comfortably forward, and imagine you fill the empty space created as you push forward (keeping your feet still) with renewed energy and a sense of a fresh start. Finish with your palms opposite your shoulders.*

Crossing Hands

THESE MOVEMENTS EXPRESS *a gathering in. Enjoy the openness of the large arm movement in step 2, and be aware of the strong, contained shape you make. Standing in this position for a few minutes as a static posture improves circulation, especially to the arms and hands, and strengthens the back. This is a defensive posture. It reaffirms a condition of central equilibrium, balance, and alignment – the body is anchored in the earth and lifted to the sky.*

1 *Leave the fingertips of both hands in their position at the end of Withdraw and Push. Draw your weight onto your right leg. This has the effect of extending the arms forward.*

2 *Fold in your hip and make a 90° turn to the right (north). Bring the toes of your left foot round to face north. Open your arms in a broad arc, palms facing north.*

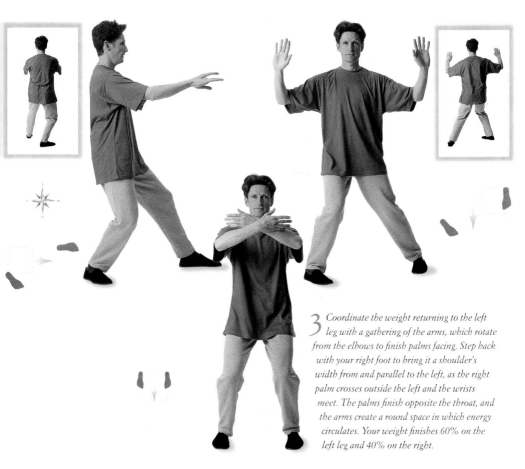

3 *Coordinate the weight returning to the left leg with a gathering of the arms, which rotate from the elbows to finish palms facing. Step back with your right foot to bring it a shoulder's width from and parallel to the left, as the right palm crosses outside the left and the wrists meet. The palms finish opposite the throat, and the arms create a round space in which energy circulates. Your weight finishes 60% on the left leg and 40% on the right.*

Embrace Tiger, Return to Mountain

START POSITION

JUSTIFYING ITS POETIC *name, Embrace Tiger, Return to Mountain is a dynamic posture. The player is called upon to move fearlessly into the path of danger to deal with an imaginary attack from the right and behind. Considering the martial application can be helpful to the performance of this posture, as it gives meaning to the turn, parry, and strike. Its develops balance and mobility and opens the hips and groin.*

1 *Sit into your left leg, dropping your right hand and turning it palm down and out. Simultaneously lift your right heel and turn right toward the northeast diagonal. Your left arm remains palm facing. Direct your attention behind you to the right.*

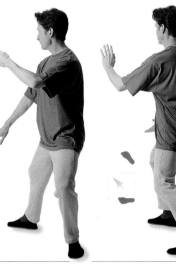

VISUALIZATION

During step 1, imagine you contact something with your right palm and the underside of your right forearm. As step 2 begins you take a step into the path of danger, and in step 3 your right arm averts it, circles, and with the left palm squeezes and pushes the threat away. Allow your mind and energy to move outward.

3 *Bring your weight forward while drawing a generous cup shape in the air with your right hand, turning it palm up near your right thigh. Drop your left elbow, turning the hand palm forward, but keeping it level with your throat.*

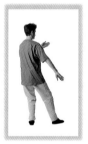

2 *Take a big step with your right foot, swinging it round to place it heel first in a bow and arrow stance on the southeast diagonal. Your right arm moves with your right leg as if attached to it. Almost all your weight remains on the back (left) leg.*

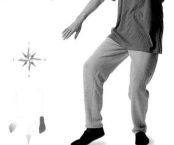

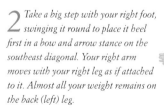

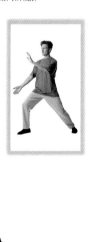

Rollback, Press, Push, and Single Whip

THIS SEQUENCE MARKS a changeover from one section of the form to another. The same movements are followed as shown on pages 68–70, but the external reference points have changed from the east-west axis to the northwest-southeast diagonal.

ROLLBACK

Here the move into Rollback differs from the page 68 version. Following step 3 of Embrace Tiger, Return to Mountain you make a small adjustment movement before progressing smoothly into step 2 and then step 3 of Rollback on page 68, aligned on the northwest-southeast diagonal.

Adjustment movement

1 *With your weight on your front (right) leg, turn to the right (south), lifting your right palm in an arc and bringing your left palm down opposite your right elbow. Focus southward, in following your arms.*

2 *Simultaneously move your weight back along the diagonal, turn your spine left, rotate your left forearm to turn the palms up, drop your right elbow to lift the hand. Finish with 70% of your weight on your back (left) leg, hips and right palm facing east, and your left fingers near your right elbow.*

3 *Continue to turn left as far as your hips will allow. Unfold your left forearm toward the north, palm up, and rest your right forearm palm down near your breastbone. Finish with 90% of your weight resting on your left leg, 10% on your right.*

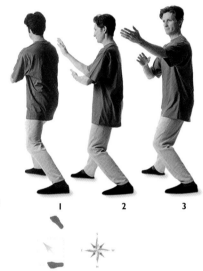

1   2   3

DIAGONAL SEQUENCE

Press

Now move smoothly into Press, following the same sequence of movements as shown on page 69, but along the diagonal.

Push

Progress without a break into Push, as shown on page 69, but this time aligning along the diagonal.

Single Whip

Glide into Single Whip as shown on pages 70–71. Finish on the diagonal, facing northwest. Pay particular attention to the final step, making sure you face the northwest diagonal and do not step all the way round to the west.

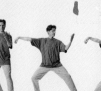

Punch Under Elbow

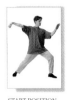

START POSITION

THROUGH DEFT FOOTWORK *this posture teaches poise, clarity, mobility, and balance in stepping. It develops warrior energy by bridging inner-centeredness with outward focus. After it you feel you can meet any challenge that comes your way. Focus on coordinating the movements and all quickly become part of a delightful whirl. At the end, focus awareness on central balance and enjoy feeling poised and focused.*

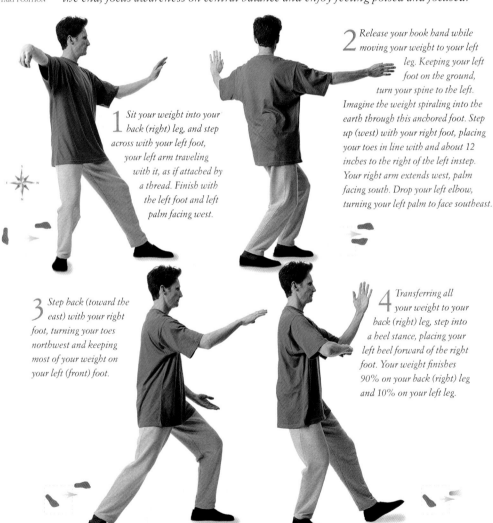

1 *Sit your weight into your back (right) leg, and step across with your left foot, your left arm traveling with it, as if attached by a thread. Finish with the left foot and left palm facing west.*

2 *Release your hook hand while moving your weight to your left leg. Keeping your left foot on the ground, turn your spine to the left. Imagine the weight spiraling into the earth through this anchored foot. Step up (west) with your right foot, placing your toes in line with and about 12 inches to the right of the left instep. Your right arm extends west, palm facing south. Drop your left elbow, turning your left palm to face southeast.*

3 *Step back (toward the east) with your right foot, turning your toes northwest and keeping most of your weight on your left (front) foot.*

4 *Transferring all your weight to your back (right) leg, step into a heel stance, placing your left heel forward of the right foot. Your weight finishes 90% on your back (right) leg and 10% on your left leg.*

Step Back to Repulse Monkey

START POSITION

THIS SPIRITED MOVE *involves testing the ground before moving the weight, and keeping a forward eye on the advancing and unpredictable imaginary monkey. This posture opens the ankle joints and exercises the Achilles tendons, which helps develop the balance and coordination needed to move backward. This posture is performed three times, first turning to the right (shown below), then to the left, then right.*

COORDINATION

Expect to struggle with the difficult coordination in this posture, particularly in step 2 where several movements happen at once. Allow your body to find its own coordination. By contast with the open shape of step 1, the body is more gathered or closed in step 2.

Right side

1 *Keeping your weight mainly on your right (back) leg and your feet still, turn your spine to the right as far as your hips allow. Extend your left arm forward (west), palm down. Release the fist as you drop your right arm, then arc it up and out to the side with the palm facing forward.*

2 *Sit deeper into your right (back) leg and, keeping the weight forward, step back with your left foot. Rest it, toes first, a shoulder's width behind and left of your right foot, aligned east-west. Meanwhile, fold your right elbow, moving the hand palm down near your right ear, and drop your left arm, rolling it toward your body, palm facing. Your right fingers point to your left palm.*

3 *Transfer your weight to your back (left) foot, bringing your right toes round to face forward (west), and drop your right elbow, so your right palm faces west opposite your right shoulder. Your left hand falls, palm up, beside your left hip. Finish with 90% of your weight on your back (left) leg and 10% on your front (right) leg, your feet parallel, a shoulder width apart, facing west. Do not lock your front leg at the knee.*

Diagonal Flying

START POSITION

DIAGONAL FLYING GENERATES *boldness. It is a celebration, an opportunity to shout fearlessly about the brilliance and passion of one's life. At the beginning, the focus is on collecting the golden light that radiated out of the body at the end of the last sequence. At the finish, let the brilliant luminescence, now gathered up, burst into the body and be anchored there by the left hand, but fly out skyward through the right.*

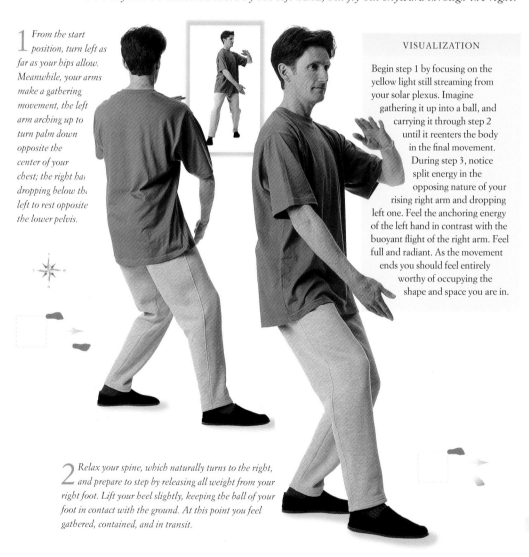

1 *From the start position, turn left as far as your hips allow. Meanwhile, your arms make a gathering movement, the left arm arching up to turn palm down opposite the center of your chest; the right hand dropping below the left to rest opposite the lower pelvis.*

VISUALIZATION

Begin step 1 by focusing on the yellow light still streaming from your solar plexus. Imagine gathering it up into a ball, and carrying it through step 2 until it reenters the body in the final movement. During step 3, notice split energy in the opposing nature of your rising right arm and dropping left one. Feel the anchoring energy of the left hand in contrast with the buoyant flight of the right arm. Feel full and radiant. As the movement ends you should feel entirely worthy of occupying the shape and space you are in.

2 *Relax your spine, which naturally turns to the right, and prepare to step by releasing all weight from your right foot. Lift your heel slightly, keeping the ball of your foot in contact with the ground. At this point you feel gathered, contained, and in transit.*

ARMS AND HANDS

As your weight moves to your right (front) leg during step 4, let your right arm fly upward, to extend palm up along the northeast diagonal. Look at the tip of your right middle finger, which is at eye level. Your left arm moves earthward toward your left thigh, palm down.

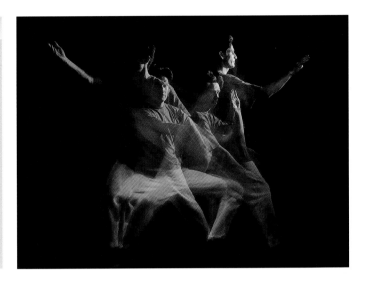

3 *Sitting deeply into your left leg, take a big step round with your right foot, placing it heel first toward the northeast.*

4 *Finish in a bow and arrow stance along the northeast diagonal, with 70% of your weight on your front (right) leg and 30% on your back leg, and your left foot aligned directly northward.*

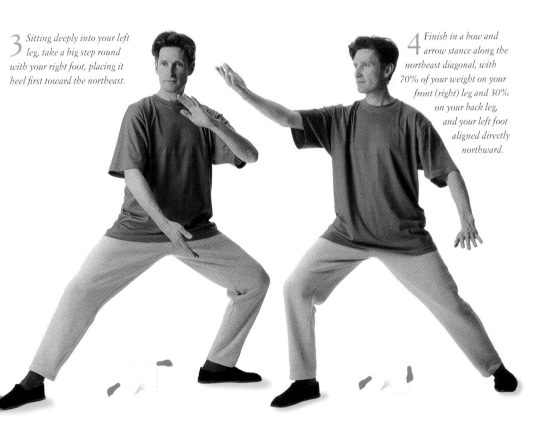

Waving Hands in Clouds

START POSITION

WAVING HANDS IS *a sequence of energy-building side steps facing north, which is repeated on the right, then on the left. Repeatedly turning the spine massages the kidneys, and successively drawing up each hand promotes energy flow, benefitting grounding and balance. Drawing energy from the solar plexus to the heart links celebrating personal power with achieving harmony with others.*

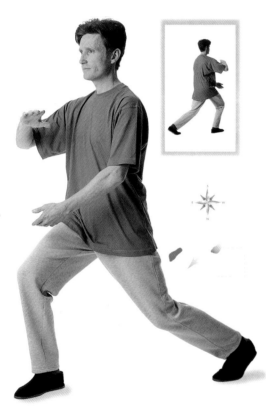

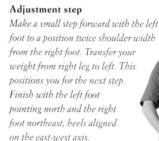

Adjustment step
Make a small step forward with the left foot to a position twice shoulder width from the right foot. Transfer your weight from right leg to left. This positions you for the next step. Finish with the left foot pointing north and the right foot northeast, heels aligned on the east-west axis.

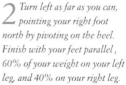

Left side
2 *Turn left as far as you can, pointing your right foot north by pivoting on the heel. Finish with your feet parallel, 60% of your weight on your left leg, and 40% on your right leg.*

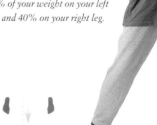

Right side
1 *Sit all your weight into your front (right) leg and, pivoting on the ball of your left foot, turn right (east). While turning, draw your right hand toward you and swivel the forearm, bringing the hand palm down opposite the center of your chest. Your left hand, palm upward, moves level with your lower pelvis. Your left leg rests behind, toes on the ground, heel lifted.*

MID-POSITION

As the weight builds in your left leg and your spine turns left in steps 2, 4, and 6, allow your left hand to rise 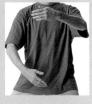 and your right hand to fall. As your body turns north, rotate your left palm to face your upper chest, and your right palm to face your lower pelvis. From this mid-position, continue turning left while slowly rotating your left palm down and your right palm up.

While you turn in steps 3 and 5, your right hand rises and your left hand falls.

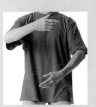 As you face north in the mid-position, both palms turn to face your body.

Left side

4 Sitting all your weight into your right leg and keeping the feet parallel, step west with the left foot, placing it twice shoulder width to the left of the right foot. Your left arm floats up, palm facing. Turn left as far as you can while dropping your right hand level with your lower pelvis and slowly turning the palm up. You finish holding a ball, left hand on top, palm down, right hand beneath, palm up; and with 60% of your weight on your left leg and 40% on your right leg.

Right side

5 Now repeat movement 3, Right Side, illustrated opposite.

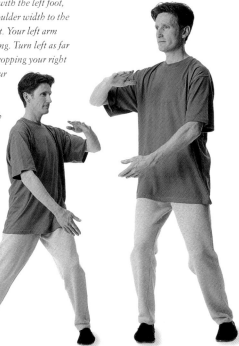

Right side

3 Sit deeply into your left leg and place your right foot parallel to it one shoulder's width away. Draw your weight from left leg to right, imagining it traveling underground, while turning your spine to the right as far as your hips comfortably allow. Finish facing northeast.

Left side

6 Repeat movement 4 Left Side, illustrated above, before proceeding to the first movement of Single Whip on the next page.

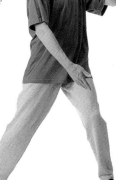

Single Whip

START POSITION

SINGLE WHIP REAPPEARS *to mark a change in direction and momentum after the foregoing sequence. In its third appearance, this posture is used to develop flowing coordination. It is energized by the ball of energy caught between the hands at the end of Waving Hands. Enjoy the sweeping arm and hand movements of step 1. Take the longest possible step into the bow and arrow stance, since it boosts the circulation.*

1 *Step directly northward with your right leg and transfer all your weight to it while turning your spine to the northeast. As you finish, your left foot rests behind, heel lifted.*

2 *Relax and turn your spine left, pivoting on the ball of your left foot. With all the balance in your right leg, take a long step west with your left foot, into a bow and arrow stance. The left palm turns to face the left shoulder.*

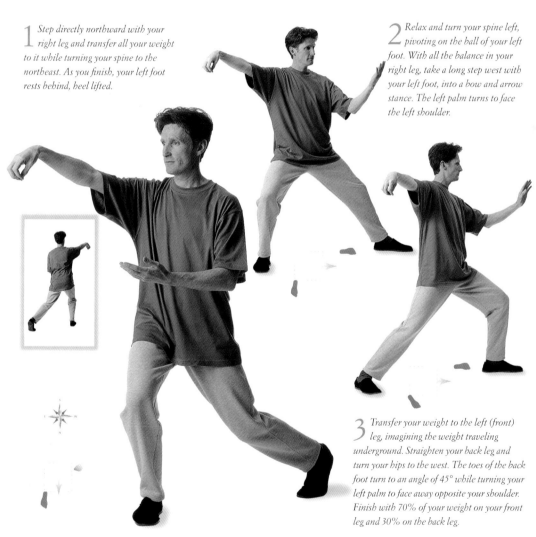

3 *Transfer your weight to the left (front) leg, imagining the weight traveling underground. Straighten your back leg and turn your hips to the west. The toes of the back foot turn to an angle of 45° while turning your left palm to face away opposite your shoulder. Finish with 70% of your weight on your front leg and 30% on the back leg.*

Squatting Single Whip

SINGLE WHIP IS *followed by a variation on itself, Squatting Single Whip. Elegant and esthetically pleasing, this is a strong, dynamic posture and a great favorite. It refreshes the body, opens the hips and pelvis, and massages the colon. It exercises the legs, boosting blood circulation and cleansing the lymph fluid that bathes the tissues. This posture is strongly cyclical – feel the drawing back in step 1 as the first quadrant of a circle, followed by moving down, forward, and up. The right hand remains in a hook shape throughout the posture.*

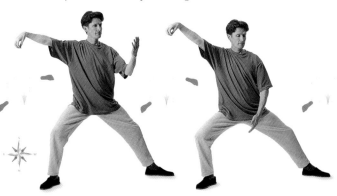

1 *Turn your right toes to the rear diagonal (northeast) and your left palm toward the center of your chest. At the same time, bring your weight back to your right leg.*

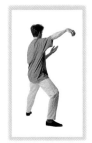

2 *Folding in the hips, drop your spine vertically as if you were squatting through your right leg, aligning your knees with your feet. Keep most of your weight back while connecting your front foot with the ground. Let your front (left) leg bend. Drop your left hand, pointing your fingers to the earth.*

3 *Turn your left toes out to the southwest, turn your hips to face west and rotate your left palm outward (facing north). Continue to drop vertically.*

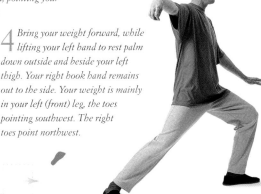

4 *Bring your weight forward, while lifting your left hand to rest palm down outside and beside your left thigh. Your right hook hand remains out to the side. Your weight is mainly in your left (front) leg, the toes pointing southwest. The right toes point northwest.*

VISUALIZATION

Squatting Single Whip is also aptly called Snake Creeps Down – during step 2, visualize yourself filling with a cascade of cosmic energy that descends from the top of your head to the base of your spine as your left hand pulls it down through your body, allowing it to earth. Imagine this force as powerfully cleansing and allow it to inspire you.

Golden Rooster Stands on One Leg

START POSITION

THIS POSTURE, PERFORMED *first on the right side and then on the left, trains the balance and develops poise. Its first step doubles as the last step of Squatting Single Whip (page 91); and the hook hand is now released as if throwing an explosive ball from the hook hand to the ground. The explosion bounces back through the right-hand fingers and returns to the sky.*

Right side

1 *Sitting your weight into your left leg, sweep your right arm downward, releasing the hook hand. Point the fingers earthward.*

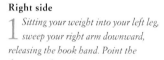

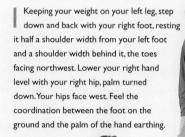

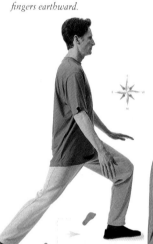

2 *Continue the arm sweep upward while lifting your right leg. Finish standing on your left leg, your right thigh parallel to the ground, the toes pointing down. Your hips and right thigh face west, your left hand has risen slightly to hip level, palm turned down, and your right-hand fingers point skyward.*

LEFT SIDE

1 Keeping your weight on your left leg, step down and back with your right foot, resting it half a shoulder width from your left foot and a shoulder width behind it, the toes facing northwest. Lower your right hand level with your right hip, palm turned down. Your hips face west. Feel the coordination between the foot on the ground and the palm of the hand earthing.

2 Drop naturally into balancing on your right leg and point the left toes west.

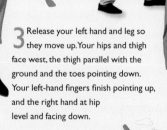

3 Release your left hand and leg so they move up. Your hips and thigh face west, the thigh parallel with the ground and the toes pointing down. Your left-hand fingers finish pointing up, and the right hand at hip level and facing down.

Separate Right Foot

START POSITION

THIS POSTURE CONTINUES *to develop balance, but takes it farther. In the last posture both legs were static during the balancing, in Separate Right Foot the body balances on the left leg and the feet are separated during a wide, swinging kick with the right foot. This movement is balanced by repeating the posture on the left side. The posture makes a dynamic link between sky and earth and the polarity of outward and inward.*

1 *Keeping most of your weight on the front (right) leg, step back with your left foot and place it facing southwest. Meanwhile, turn to the front right diagonal as if catching something between your arms. Look along the diagonal, gazing upward slightly.*

2 *Moving your weight to your back (left) leg, pull down with your arms.*

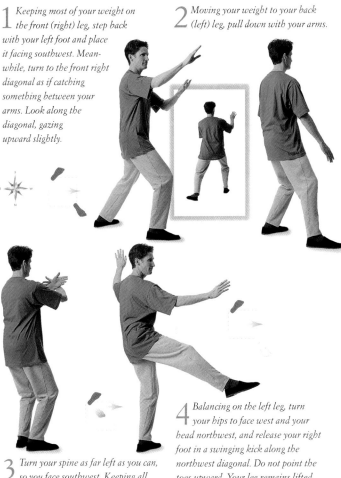

CROSSING HANDS

As you move one foot next to the other during step 2, make a full circle with your arms, finishing with the hands crossed, right hand on the outside, opposite your throat. In Separate Left Foot (page 94) cross your left hand over your right hand. Direct your awareness clearly inward and feel your alignment into the earth.

HANDS AND ARMS

Just before you kick in step 3, open your arms, turning the palms outwards. In Separate Right Foot align the right arm with the right leg just above shoulder height, extending the left arm out to the side for balance. In Separate Left Foot align your left arm with your left leg and extend your right arm out to the side.

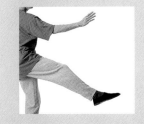

3 *Turn your spine as far left as you can, so you face southwest. Keeping all your weight on the left leg, rest your right foot, heel lifted, beside the left.*

4 *Balancing on the left leg, turn your hips to face west and your head northwest, and release your right foot in a swinging kick along the northwest diagonal. Do not point the toes upward. Your leg remains lifted, thigh parallel to the floor, knee bent, toes pointing downward.*

Separate Left Foot

BEGIN THIS MOVEMENT *with the same pulling down motion as in Separate Right Foot; then reverse all of the movements. This posture stimulates circulation and increases mental dexterity, with a shifting of awareness inward and then outward. While aligning with the left diagonal, accompany the movement of your "catching" arms by focusing awareness to the southwest.*

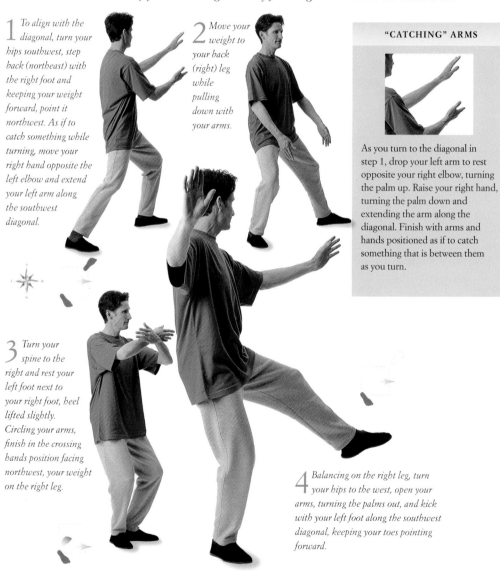

1 *To align with the diagonal, turn your hips southwest, step back (northeast) with the right foot and keeping your weight forward, point it northwest. As if to catch something while turning, move your right hand opposite the left elbow and extend your left arm along the southwest diagonal.*

2 *Move your weight to your back (right) leg while pulling down with your arms.*

"CATCHING" ARMS

As you turn to the diagonal in step 1, drop your left arm to rest opposite your right elbow, turning the palm up. Raise your right hand, turning the palm down and extending the arm along the diagonal. Finish with arms and hands positioned as if to catch something that is between them as you turn.

3 *Turn your spine to the right and rest your left foot next to your right foot, heel lifted slightly. Circling your arms, finish in the crossing hands position facing northwest, your weight on the right leg.*

4 *Balancing on the right leg, turn your hips to the west, open your arms, turning the palms out, and kick with your left foot along the southwest diagonal, keeping your toes pointing forward.*

Brush Knee and Push, Needles at Sea Bottom

START POSITION

THE SEVEN POSTURES *on the following pages are the variation in the form created by Dr. Chi Chiang-tao (see pages 62–63). The variation begins with a slightly different version of Brush Knee and Push, which acts as a breather. Needles at Sea Bottom massages the colon, stimulating it to function more efficiently.*

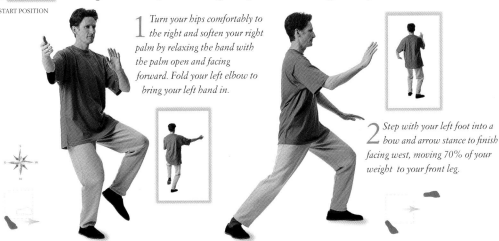

1 *Turn your hips comfortably to the right and soften your right palm by relaxing the hand with the palm open and facing forward. Fold your left elbow to bring your left hand in.*

2 *Step with your left foot into a bow and arrow stance to finish facing west, moving 70% of your weight to your front leg.*

NEEDLES AT SEA BOTTOM

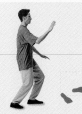
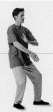
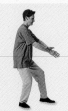

1 Step with your right foot to rest it just behind the left, while transferring your weight to the left leg. Direct your mind out and forward to focus it on what you are going to do next.

2 Move your weight to the right (rear) leg, turn a little to the right, and bring your left palm next to your right elbow.

3 Release your left foot and place it in a cat stance. Straighten your hips toward the front (west), send your right hand down diagonally away from you, and slide your left palm down onto your right wrist.

4 Keeping 90% of your weight seated in your right leg, fold in your hips by bending your knees and inclining your spine forward. Keep your spine aligned from the coccyx to the head.

Iron Fan

THIS STRONG POSTURE *grows like a tree, with a rising momentum in the form of a trunk and a spreading, branchlike shape. It imparts strength, focus, and warrior energy. As you follow step 2, let the energy of the posture fill your body and extend along your spreading arms. As you deepen your stance, extend your arms. Anchored firmly by your legs, yet focused on the space where your right-hand fingers are projecting, allow the warrior in your soul to flood your body.*

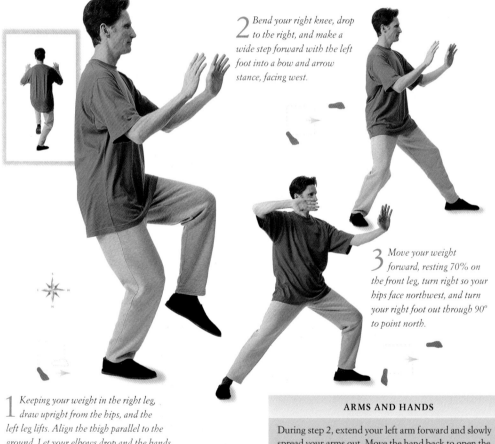

2 Bend your right knee, drop to the right, and make a wide step forward with the left foot into a bow and arrow stance, facing west.

3 Move your weight forward, resting 70% on the front leg, turn right so your hips face northwest, and turn your right foot out through 90° to point north.

1 Keeping your weight in the right leg, draw upright from the hips, and the left leg lifts. Align the thigh parallel to the ground. Let your elbows drop and the hands float and rest, quietly alert, in front of the body. Maintain internal equilibrium while feeling the posture's upward growth.

ARMS AND HANDS

During step 2, extend your left arm forward and slowly spread your arms out. Move the hand back to open the palm fully toward the right diagonal. During step 3 draw your right hand back, rotating the forearm outward and bringing it parallel to the ground. Your right hand finishes beside your face, palm facing out.

Turn Body, Chop, and Push

START POSITION

THIS COORDINATED DANCE *between hands and feet expresses the energy of the cosmos and the earth. The fist you make with your right hand draws power from the earth, while your left hand draws energy from the sky, and the two fuel the forward-moving fist and the push at the finish. The posture teaches coordination between stepping, weight shifts, hands, and feet.*

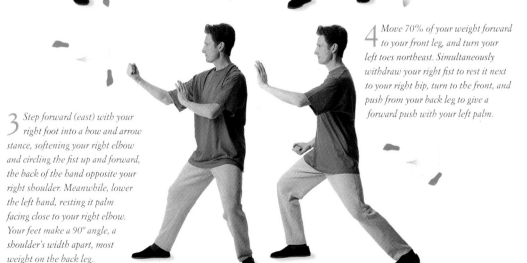

1 *Turn to the right (north) as far as your hips allow, bringing most of your weight into your right leg. Follow it with your left foot, which pivots on the heel to finish pointing north.*

2 *Keep turning right to face northeast and move most of your weight back to the left leg. Lift the right heel and pivot on the ball of the foot. Unfold your elbow and drop the fist, resting it outside and next to your right thigh.*

HANDS AND ARMS

As you turn in step 1, bring your left hand above your head, palm away. Lower your right forearm to chest level, making a fist of the right hand, facing down.

4 *Move 70% of your weight forward to your front leg, and turn your left toes northeast. Simultaneously withdraw your right fist to rest it next to your right hip, turn to the front, and push from your back leg to give a forward push with your left palm.*

3 *Step forward (east) with your right foot into a bow and arrow stance, softening your right elbow and circling the fist up and forward, the back of the hand opposite your right shoulder. Meanwhile, lower the left hand, resting it palm facing close to your right elbow. Your feet make a 90° angle, a shoulder's width apart, most weight on the back leg.*

Bring Down and Punch(2)

THIS MOVE LINKS *Turn Body, Chop, and Push with Punch and has a strong grounding effect. Begin by reaching up with your right hand in one large rolling movement. The bringing down is expressed as the right hand falls. End by storing energy in the hui yin energy center in the lower pelvis.*

1 *Keep your weight on your front leg, open your right hip and turn left slightly to face north. Simultaneously release your fist and send your right hand up to shoulder level, palm facing left and fingers pointing forward.*

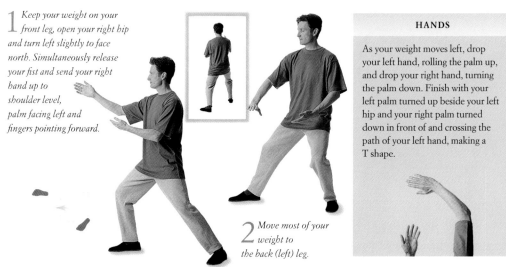

2 *Move most of your weight to the back (left) leg.*

HANDS

As your weight moves left, drop your left hand, rolling the palm up, and drop your right hand, turning the palm down. Finish with your left palm turned up beside your left hip and your right palm turned down in front of and crossing the path of your left hand, making a T shape.

PUNCH (2)

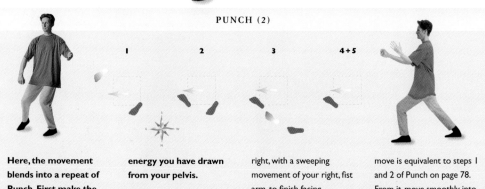

Here, the movement blends into a repeat of Punch. First make the adjustment move, then follow steps 3, 4, 5, and 6 from Punch on pages 78–79. Focus the root

energy you have drawn from your pelvis.

Adjustment move
Release your right foot to step, make a fist with your right hand, and turn to the

right, with a sweeping movement of your right, fist arm, to finish facing southeast. Now move directly into step 3 of Punch on page 78, and follow with steps 4–6 on page 79. This adjustment

move is equivalent to steps 1 and 2 of Punch on page 78. From it, move smoothly into steps 3–5 shown here. The arm movements are exactly the same as in steps 3–6 of Punch on pages 78–79.

Kick with Heel

A PHASE OF EMPTINESS *occurs at the beginning of Kick With Heel, following the fullness of the energy held after the punch that ends the previous posture. As you begin, experience total emptiness. Step 2 returns you to a fullness rooted in the Earth's center. The right heel kick comes at the end from an inward gathering, centering, and focusing. Kick with Heel improves coordination between mind and body.*

START POSITION

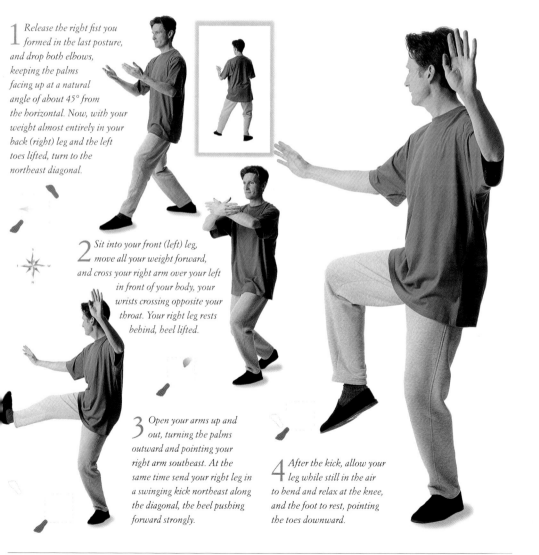

1 *Release the right fist you formed in the last posture, and drop both elbows, keeping the palms facing up at a natural angle of about 45° from the horizontal. Now, with your weight almost entirely in your back (right) leg and the left toes lifted, turn to the northeast diagonal.*

2 *Sit into your front (left) leg, move all your weight forward, and cross your right arm over your left in front of your body, your wrists crossing opposite your throat. Your right leg rests behind, heel lifted.*

3 *Open your arms up and out, turning the palms outward and pointing your right arm southeast. At the same time send your right leg in a swinging kick northeast along the diagonal, the heel pushing forward strongly.*

4 *After the kick, allow your leg while still in the air to bend and relax at the knee, and the foot to rest, pointing the toes downward.*

EALING TERTIARY COLLEGE
LEARNING RESOURCE CENTRE - EALING GREEN

Brush Right Knee and Push

*KICK WITH HEEL is followed by Brush Right Knee and Push, here in its role as a breather
between two sequences of postures. Its fourth appearance in the form mirrors the version
on page 95 exactly. Remember to be aware of the drawing-in momentum of the first
part of the posture, and the sending-out feeling during the second.*

1 *Keeping your balance on the left leg,
turn left until your hips face northeast,
folding your right arm and softening your
left palm so it faces forward. Your right
hand comes to rest palm down opposite
the center of your chest.*

2 *Step with your right foot to lead into
a right bow and arrow stance facing
directly east and with 70% of your weight
in your front (right) foot and 30% on your
back leg.*

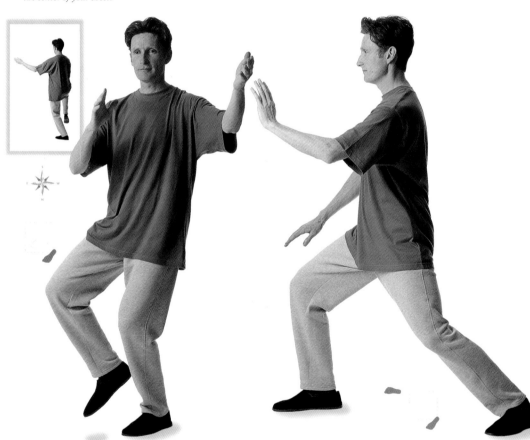

Brush Left Knee and Punch Downward

START POSITION

AT THIS POINT, *where the Cheng Man-ch'ing variation and the Chi Chiang-tao versions of the form rejoin, postures from earlier in the form reappear, marking the beginning of a change. First, the Brush Knee posture is expressed again, but this time as a punch instead of a push. Brush Left Knee And Punch Downward develops a sense of solid strength. It can transform the energy of indecision into direction.*

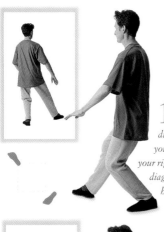

1 *Turn right to the southeast diagonal, anchor on your rear leg and place your right foot on the diagonal. Drop your left hand as the weight moves back.*

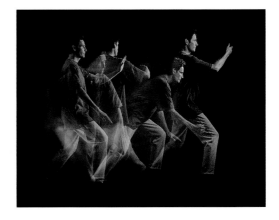

4 *As your weight moves, the downward-facing palm of your moving left hand clears your left knee to finish forward. Powered by your straightening back leg, punch down, then along. Finish facing east with your spine inclined and 80% of your weight on your front (left) leg and 20% on your back leg.*

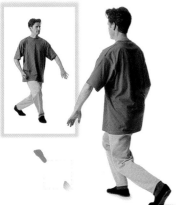

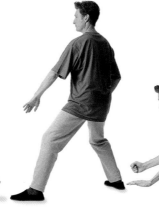

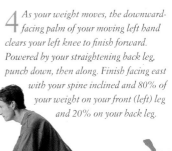

2 *Sit your weight into your right leg and rest your left foot behind, heel lifted. Form a fist with your left hand as the weight moves into the front leg.*

3 *Step east with your left foot and transfer your weight forward, forming a bow and arrow stance.*

Ward Off Right

THIS POSTURE IS *a repeat of Ward Off Right on page 67, but it originates at a different point. Where the first Ward Off Right grew out of a contained solidity, this one comes directly from a solid commitment. While bringing your weight forward during step 2, feel the wave of Ward Off energy pass from the hui yin center in the lower pelvis, up through your body and in front of it, to the level of your throat. Ward Off Right moves into Rollback, then Press, Push, and Single Whip, marking the end of the second sequence of postures.*

1 Turn to the left and place your foot on the diagonal. Release the fist and draw your right hand back and in with a sense of gathering and raising. Your left fingers and hips point northeast.

2 Drop your weight onto your front (left) leg and lift your right heel, while moving your right hand up and forward.

3 Step with your right foot into a bow and arrow stance facing east. Your right hand rests, palm facing, at throat level; the left fingers point to the right palm. Your weight finishes 70% on the front leg, 30% on the back leg.

PRIMARY POSTURES

Rollback and Press both come from a pattern of spinal movements. Push intercepts this pattern. Single Whip occurs five times in the Chen Man-ch'ing form, each marking a change in direction and momentum.

ROLLBACK – See page 68

PRESS – See page 69

PUSH – See page 69

SINGLE WHIP – See page 70

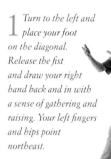

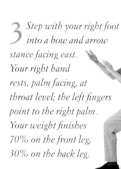

Fair Lady Weaves the Shuttle (1)

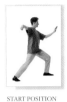

START POSITION

THIS POSTURE HAS *four positions that repeat, two on the left and two on the right. The first is illustrated here and the second, third, and fourth on the following pages. Each non-cardinal direction is visited in counterclockwise order – northeast, northwest, southwest, and southeast – against which the body weaves a web of movements in a delightful play. A complete circle is covered in the Fair Lady sequence of postures.*

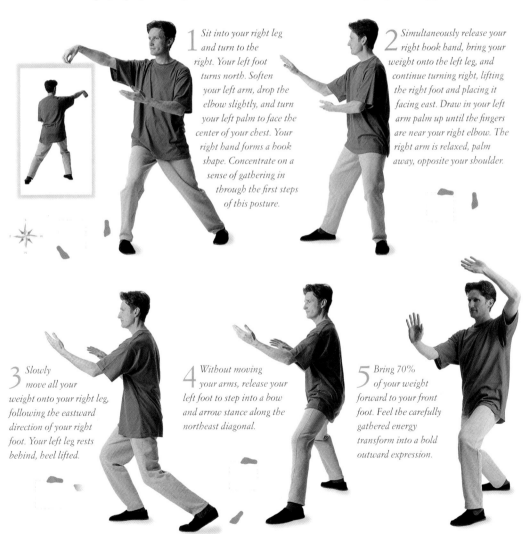

1 *Sit into your right leg and turn to the right. Your left foot turns north. Soften your left arm, drop the elbow slightly, and turn your left palm to face the center of your chest. Your right hand forms a hook shape. Concentrate on a sense of gathering in through the first steps of this posture.*

2 *Simultaneously release your right hook hand, bring your weight onto the left leg, and continue turning right, lifting the right foot and placing it facing east. Draw in your left arm palm up until the fingers are near your right elbow. The right arm is relaxed, palm away, opposite your shoulder.*

3 *Slowly move all your weight onto your right leg, following the eastward direction of your right foot. Your left leg rests behind, heel lifted.*

4 *Without moving your arms, release your left foot to step into a bow and arrow stance along the northeast diagonal.*

5 *Bring 70% of your weight forward to your front foot. Feel the carefully gathered energy transform into a bold outward expression.*

Fair Lady Weaves the Shuttle (2, 3, and 4)

START POSITION

THE FIRST POSITION *in the Fair Lady sequence of postures (page 103) moves without a break into the second position, below. The Fair Lady links the crown energy center to the heart center, encouraging communion with the surrounding space. Practiced outdoors, these postures encourage communication with nature. Indoors, they might clear space or the atmosphere in a room or in a new house.*

Fair Lady Weaves the Shuttle (2)

1 Move your weight to the right leg, and pivoting on the left heel, turn the left foot 90°. Rotating the hips southeast, roll your left arm down and toward you so the palm faces your throat, and roll your right hand toward the solar plexus, turning up the palm.

2 Bring all your weight onto your back leg while turning right, lifting the right heel to adjust the foot's position. Move the right foot about 9 inches to the right and place it on the ground facing south.

3 Move your weight to the right leg, lift your left heel, and pivot on the ball of your left foot until your hips face southwest. The right foot points south and the left rests behind, heel lifted, aligned on the diagonal.

4 Move your weight back to your left foot which, with your hips, faces southwest. Slide your right foot toward it. Turning your spine to the right, move your right foot back past the left foot along the northwest diagonal, placing it heel first, toes pointing northwest. Your hips face west.

5 Bring 70% of your weight to the right leg, turn your hips northwest, and your left toes west, finishing in a bow and arrow stance along the northwest diagonal. Roll your right arm above your head, turning the palm north; the left hand pushes forward opposite the shoulder along the diagonal.

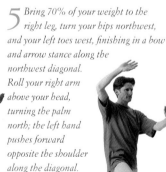

CHANGING HANDS

As your weight moves back in step 2 of Fair Lady 2 and 4, roll your left hand, palm toward the right, and rest it opposite your solar plexus, palm away. Drop your right elbow and float the right hand up, passing the descending left palm, to rest it opposite the center of your chest. Your left fingers point to the right palm and remain there during steps 3 and 4.

FAIR LADY WEAVES THE SHUTTLE (3)

1 Bring your weight to your back leg while rolling your left palm to face your solar plexus. Drop your right elbow, bringing your right arm to face palm away opposite your right shoulder. Release your right foot to place it pointing west, keeping your weight back.

2 Transfer your weight to your right leg, raising your left hand to face your throat. The right arm drops and faces palm away, and the fingers point at the left palm.

3 Step with your left foot into a bow and arrow stance along the southwest diagonal. As your weight moves to your left leg, raise your left arm and roll the palm out and up. Your right hand pushes forward. Notice the link between the left hand meeting the sky and the right hand sending outward.

Fair Lady Weaves the Shuttle (4)

1 Move your weight to your right leg, then pivoting on your left heel turn the foot 90° to point northwest, and turn your hips northwest. As you turn, roll your left arm down toward your throat, and your right hand toward your solar plexus, palm up.

2 Bring all your weight to your back leg while turning right, lifting the right heel to adjust the foot. Meanwhile, your hands change as shown in the box (opposite). Move the right foot about 9 inches to the right and place it facing north.

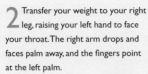

3 Transfer your weight to your right leg, lift the left heel, and turning the hips northeast, pivot on your left foot. Your right foot points to the north, your left foot resting behind it, heel lifted, is aligned along the northeast-southwest diagonal.

4 Move your weight back to your left foot, which, with your hips, faces northeast. Slide your right foot toward it. Turning your spine right, move your right foot back past the left foot along the diagonal, placing it heel first, facing southeast. Your hips face east.

5 Bring 70% of your weight to the right leg, turning your hips southeast and your left toes to the east, adopting a bow and arrow stance along the southeast diagonal. Simultaneously roll your left arm down toward your throat, and your right hand toward your solar plexus, turning the palm up. Roll your right arm above the head, turning the palm southward; and push your left hand forward opposite the left shoulder.

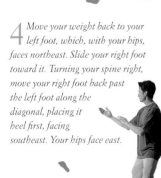

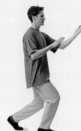

105

Ward Off Left

START POSITION

THE MOVES ON *these two pages mark the end of the Fair Lady sequence of postures and the start of a series of postures that ends the form. Ward Off Left ends as on page 66, but it emerges from the movements woven through the four positions of Fair Lady on the preceding pages, and although it concentrates on gathering in, it has a different feeling, delivering a sense of containment and completion.*

1 *Keeping your weight on your front leg, draw the right foot round to point east. Drop the left hand and roll it palm up to rest opposite the lower pelvis; and rest the right hand palm down opposite the center of your chest. At the end, your hands hold a ball.*

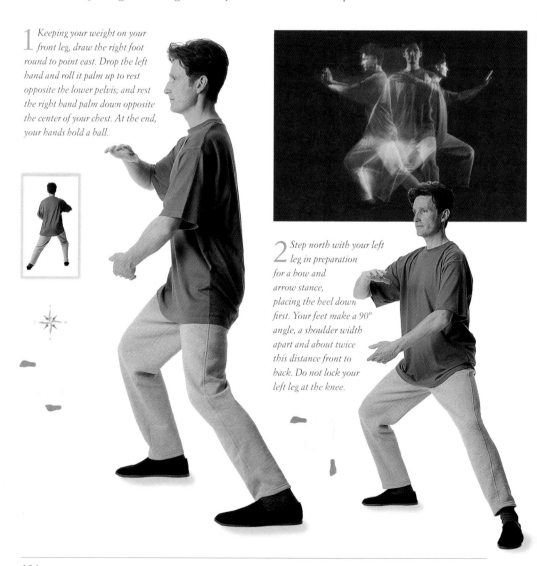

2 *Step north with your left leg in preparation for a bow and arrow stance, placing the heel down first. Your feet make a 90° angle, a shoulder width apart and about twice this distance front to back. Do not lock your left leg at the knee.*

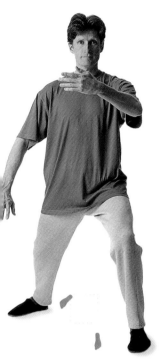

WARD OFF RIGHT

This repeat of the posture shown on page 67 energizes the whole body by drawing the creative sexual energy of Ward Off through it.

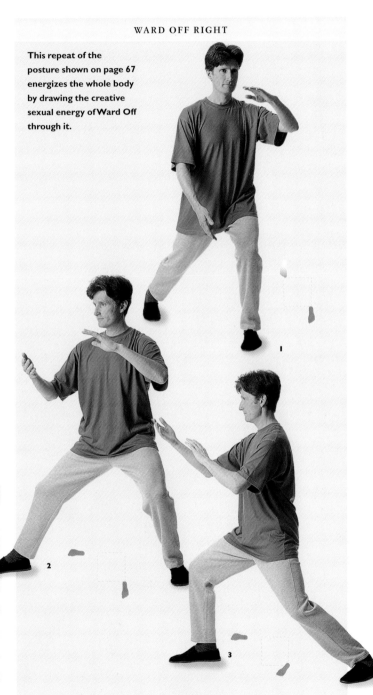

3 *Transfer your weight forward, while raising the left arm and lowering the right hand. Pushing down with your back foot straightens your back leg, turns your body north, and turns the toes of the back foot 45° to face northeast. Finish with 70% of your weight on the back leg and 30% on the front.*

VISUALIZATION

The sense of gathering in step 1 comes from the magic woven by the Fair Lady postures. Imagine holding the Earth in your hands, and in step 2, filling with the energy of the primary posture Ward Off, which comes from holding the world. Note how the posture's final shape feels contained, and the right hand acts as an anchor into the earth.

Squatting Single Whip

START POSITION

IN ITS SECOND *appearance in the form Squatting Single Whip (also called Snake Creeps Down) brings cosmic energy from the sky to earth through the body. At the end it merges into a new posture with a strong, warrior-like position, called Step Forward to the Seven Stars, perhaps a reference to a constellation – the Big Dipper or Plow which has seven stars. The energy of Squatting Single Whip fills the Seven Stars.*

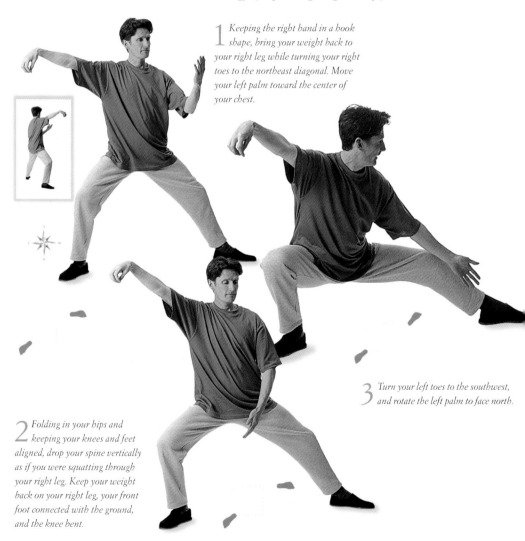

1 *Keeping the right hand in a hook shape, bring your weight back to your right leg while turning your right toes to the northeast diagonal. Move your left palm toward the center of your chest.*

2 *Folding in your hips and keeping your knees and feet aligned, drop your spine vertically as if you were squatting through your right leg. Keep your weight back on your right leg, your front foot connected with the ground, and the knee bent.*

3 *Turn your left toes to the southwest, and rotate the left palm to face north.*

Step Forward to the Seven Stars and Step Back to Ride Tiger

START POSITION

THE POSITION OF *the body in the first posture resembles the Plow constellation, with the right foot, knee, and hip, and the two elbows and fists forming a similar pattern whose attributes are strength, focus, and integrity. The role of the second posture is to ready the player to meet any adversary – dealing in an impartial manner with the need of the moment, defusing and earthing the threatening tiger energy.*

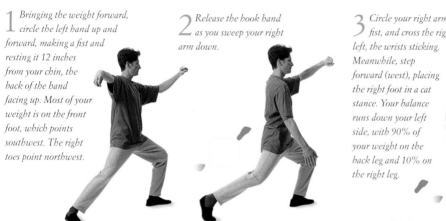

1 *Bringing the weight forward, circle the left hand up and forward, making a fist and resting it 12 inches from your chin, the back of the hand facing up. Most of your weight is on the front foot, which points southwest. The right toes point northwest.*

2 *Release the hook hand as you sweep your right arm down.*

3 *Circle your right arm up forming a fist, and cross the right wrist over the left, the wrists sticking. Meanwhile, step forward (west), placing the right foot in a cat stance. Your balance runs down your left side, with 90% of your weight on the back leg and 10% on the right leg.*

STEP BACK TO RIDE TIGER

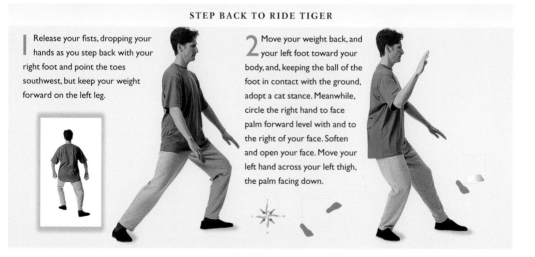

1 Release your fists, dropping your hands as you step back with your right foot and point the toes southwest, but keep your weight forward on the left leg.

2 Move your weight back, and your left foot toward your body, and, keeping the ball of the foot in contact with the ground, adopt a cat stance. Meanwhile, circle the right hand to face palm forward level with and to the right of your face. Soften and open your face. Move your left hand across your left thigh, the palm facing down.

Turn and Sweep Lotus

START POSITION

TURN AND SWEEP LOTUS, *with its swirling movement and explosive sweep-kick at the end, is like shouting an enjoyable "Hey!" in celebration of the form. The speed of the sweep brings a relief from the steady rhythm of the other postures. The difficult turn in this posture works well when the mind and body form a downward, inward spiral. This posture therefore improves balance and encourages good coordination.*

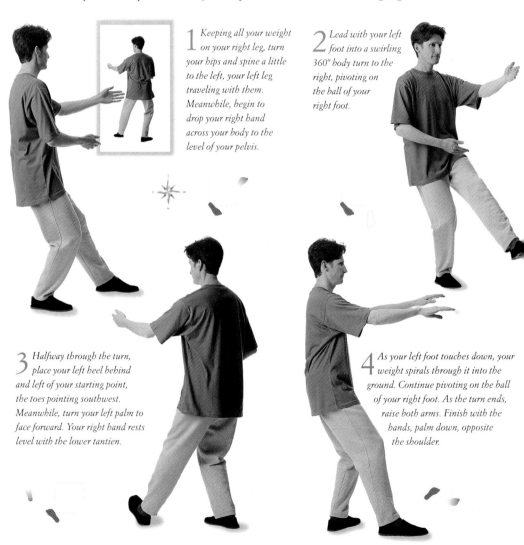

1 *Keeping all your weight on your right leg, turn your hips and spine a little to the left, your left leg traveling with them. Meanwhile, begin to drop your right hand across your body to the level of your pelvis.*

2 *Lead with your left foot into a swirling 360° body turn to the right, pivoting on the ball of your right foot.*

3 *Halfway through the turn, place your left heel behind and left of your starting point, the toes pointing southwest. Meanwhile, turn your left palm to face forward. Your right hand rests level with the lower tantien.*

4 *As your left foot touches down, your weight spirals through it into the ground. Continue pivoting on the ball of your right foot. As the turn ends, raise both arms. Finish with the hands, palm down, opposite the shoulder.*

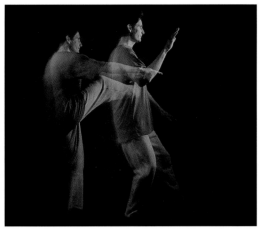

5 Anchor firmly in your left leg and lift your right knee, moving it left.

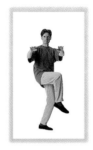

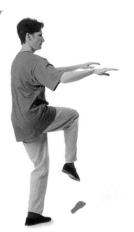

6 Sweep your right leg to the right across your body in a downward-curving arc.

7 Concentrate on lifting your knee as high as you can during the kick, without losing your balance.

8 Bring your leg back to the center and rest it, knee lifted and foot pointing down. The arms remain comfortably extended. Finish with your left foot pointing southwest and your body facing toward the west.

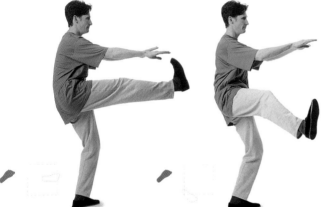

VISUALIZATION

Learning how to break the pattern of "challenge equals stress" involves understanding how to drop the center of gravity in a challenging situation. The secret is to direct the attention inward at the beginning of the posture, and to visualize the center of gravity spiraling downward through the spinning right foot, and becoming a smooth pirouette with the transfer of weight to the left foot.

THE KICK

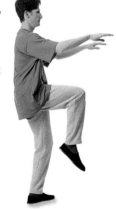

As it passes under your hands during the kick in step 6, let your right foot clip the fingers of both hands with a smacking sound. In order to make contact between foot and hand, you need to mobilize your hips and keep your knee high. This might take some practice, and if you find it impossible at first, concentrate on lifting your knee as high as you can without losing your balance.

Bend Bow to Shoot Tiger

BEND BOW TO *Shoot Tiger is the final posture in the form with a warrior stance and calls for disciplined movements and steady rhythm. Its strong downward momentum restores a deep connection with the earth, from which comes the warrior stance at the end. It has a strong grounding effect and can give a feeling of strength, focus, and integrity. The posture moves into Punch, which has the same slow, even tempo.*

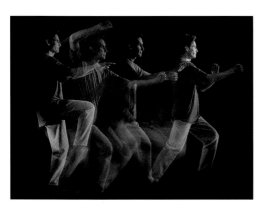

VISUALIZATION

Join the downward momentum of step 1 with your eyes, focusing on the earthing effect of this part of the move. Keep your spirit lifted. During step 2 your hands form fists softly but definitely, as if drawing on the energy of the earth. Feel the distance between the fists increase as the movement progresses, as if you were stretching a bow, and how the left fist in particular extends away from your strongly anchored body.

1 *Drop your spine and arms as you turn to the right, placing the right foot on the northwest diagonal. Your arms sweep down, palms facing down as if they were bringing something to earth. The left leg bends at the knee to allow the spine to drop. Keep your weight mainly on the back leg.*

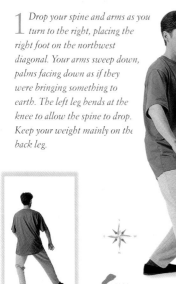

2 *Continue to turn right as you form fists with both hands and circle them forward and up. The left foot points southwest; the right foot is a shoulder's width from it and forward in a stance to the northwest. Start to bring your weight forward, your fists rising.*

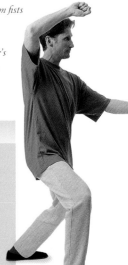

HANDS

Move 70% of your weight well forward to your front (right) foot during step 2, while raising your right fist level with the top of your head. Continue sending your left fist forward to finish comfortably opposite your solar plexus. If you were holding a pencil in your left hand, it would lean at an angle of 45° to the perpendicular.

Punch (3)

THIS POSTURE FIRST *appeared on pages 78–79, but it emerges from a different place, so the movements in the first two steps are different. Releasing the left fist in step 1 gives a sense of letting go of Bend Bow To Shoot Tiger. The downward movement gives the impression of storing, as if you were gathering the warrior energy encountered through the form. From step 3 follow the movements shown on page 79, putting heart and soul into the punch in step 6.*

1 *Sit into your right leg and release your left fist.*

2 *Step back with your left foot, and bringing your weight back, turn to the left. Rotate your left hand palm up while dropping it to rest beside your left thigh, and tilt your right fist (palm down, were it open) in front of your left fingers. Pivot on the ball of your right foot to face southwest.*

3 *From step 2, move into step 3 of the version of Punch on page 78, and continue through to step 6.*

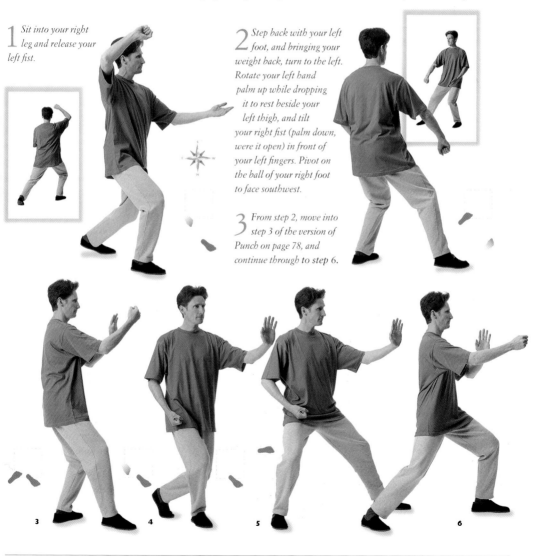

3   4   5   6

Withdraw and Push and Crossing Hands

TWO POSTURES FROM *early on – Withdraw and Push and Crossing Hands – recur, but although the same movements are repeated in the same order, the story woven by these two postures differs slightly from the tale they told earlier on, because here they are concerned with the form's conclusion. They deliver a sense of integrating and calling together. Start by following the steps for Withdraw and Push on page 80.*

1 *Gently releasing the fist you formed in the last posture, move into the first step of Withdraw and Push, then follow steps 2 and 3.*

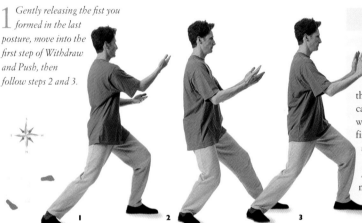

1

2

3

VISUALIZATION

Compare the feeling of your open, empty hand with your closed fist and imagine dandelion seeds blown from your hand by the wind, or some other image that carries a sense of release, such as a white dove flying from your fingers. As you withdraw, maintain a sense that you are clearing the space of the story of the form. And as you push, see the movement as a wish to fill your life with clear, positive energy.

CROSSING HANDS

This final posture restores equilibrium. Follow the steps shown in Crossing Hands on page 81, concentrating on the strong, contained shape your body makes and its alignment, anchored in the earth and lifted to the sky. Open up to the universe before creating the final seal as your wrists cross.

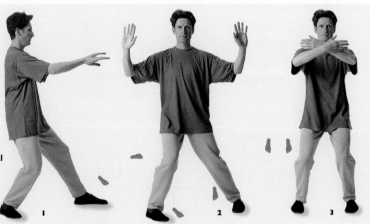

1

2

3

Completion

SO MUCH ENERGY is held in the final moment. Like the last note in an opera, the sound and the energy of the form need to remain clear and linger after the movements are completed, leaving a sustained note of beauty and dignity. This moment deserves to be savored so that the energy so carefully built up through each posture is not lost but stored and nurtured. The form should create a rich treasury of energy on which body and soul can feed. As your hands come down, feel this as a final clearing of the form and of your space. Finish with an acknowledgment of the reality of your situation: you are simply a human standing on the earth.

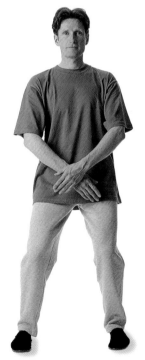

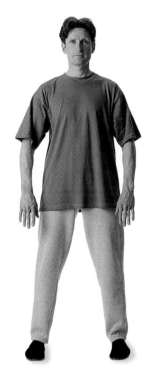

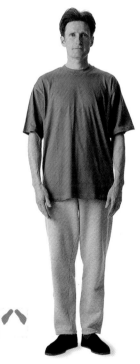

1 *Drop your hands slowly to your sides. As you do so, reverse the relative positions of your hands so that the left hand, which is inside as Crossing Hands finishes, passes over the outside of the right hand.*

2 *As you move your hands, straighten your legs and stand naturally.*

3 *Carefully draw in your right heel and then your left, ending the form in the position in which you began it.*

Branching Out

TAI CHI IS *a rich art with wide applications. Many people practice all their lives for their health, while some take up the complementary art of qigung. Both systems work to maximize energy, reduce stress, and maintain health, but whereas qigung concentrates on solo practice, working with a partner is central to tai chi. Partnerwork is a way of applying the solo form of tai chi to everyday life. It creates many different situations between two people based on a rhythm of pushing and yielding, from which it becomes possible to perceive how one relates to other people. The principles of partner practice have wider applications, for they are what make tai chi a martial art.*

The tai chi form has long been part of the daily routine for many people concerned with strengthening the body and the immune system. Performed regularly, it keeps the joints mobile, improves blood circulation, and stimulates breathing; it in addition, can improve concentration, reduce anxiety and depression, and dispel insomnia. The cultivation of health is the central principle of qigung (also written "chigung" and "chi kung," see page 122), an art that is very close to tai chi but that focuses almost exclusively on stimulating the flow of chi, or life energy,

around the body through exercise and control of the breath. Qigung develops strength, vitality, and stamina and can be effective in relieving chronic illness, improving debilitating disorders, and healing old or new injuries.

Tai chi differs from qigung in a number of ways, foremost of which is the practice of exercising with a

BELOW *Tai chi partner practice offers great potential for self-development and transformation, as this sequence shows. 1, 2 & 3, holding your space teaches confidence and trust. A collapsed body shape is easily upset.*

partner. The richness of the art of tai chi can never be experienced without exploring partnerwork (see pages 118–19). Partnerwork both supports and strengthens tai chi practice by encouraging people to think about how they give, listen, and receive. This process enables them to pinpoint personal difficulties that prevent them from interacting effectively with other people. In searching for ways of overcoming problems in a class, people find a transformation taking place in their reactions to and relationships with other people.

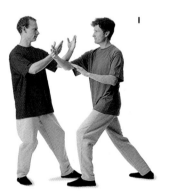
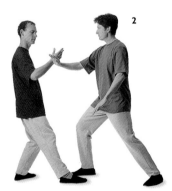
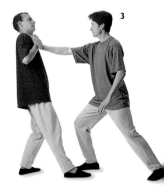

WORKING TOGETHER

Partnerwork plays an important role in helping people to affirm and put into perspective the qualities they are developing in their solo practice. It also helps to nurture ways of thought and action that are useful and relevant in day-to-day meetings with others. A great deal of life energy is required in everyday situations and tai chi partnerwork is designed to train people to use it wisely. While negotiating with people at work, dealing with an official, chatting with a friend, or having an argument with someone, it is important to be able to listen, respond, and hold one's space.

This process is exactly what happens in tai chi pair practice. Exchanges take place between partners in which each receives a push and gives a push in return. During this process of physical contact, patterns and habits of behavior reveal themselves. Some people, for example, tense up because they feel threatened by a push from a partner. By learning to relax physically and to listen to another person through the medium of touch, they are able to deal with the situation without

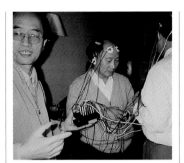

ABOVE *A Chinese qigung master takes part in a psycho-physiological experiment to measure the external emission of qi or life energy from his body.*

stress and to respond more freely. This carries through into their daily relationships with other people.

On the other hand, some people dislike having to push a partner in a tai chi exercise. This inhibition can be overcome by learning to see a push as an opportunity for the partner to respond. Some students find this a liberating experience and feel happier speaking their mind in situations where they have always felt disregarded. This is just one way in which tai chi partner practice can have a transforming effect.

BELOW *4, 5 & 6, Tai chi develops the ability to respond while holding your space.*

The following pages explore the many branches of tai chi. Those who take up tai chi for health reasons are sometimes surprised to learn that every movement, every posture in the form has an application as an evasive or attacking movement in a martial situation. There are defensive withdrawals and evasive rollbacks which, in a fight, can be used to evade a blow and regain control before moving into an attacking kick or punch. Partnerwork is an important part of practice for anyone who takes up tai chi as a fighting art, and page 120 shows pair forms relevant to its martial application.

Tai chi is not only an ancient "empty hand" art, it extends to a number of ancient weapons arts. Page 121 illustrates forms devised to develop expertise in the use of the staff and the three traditional tai chi weapons: the spear, the long sword, and the broad sword. Even the peaceful, inward-directed qigung (pages 122–23) once had a martial application in the associated neigung, an approach to the art aimed at building physical and mental resistance to blows when fighting out on a battlefield.

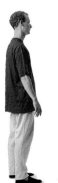
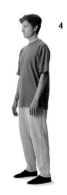

4

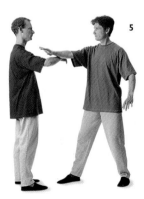

5

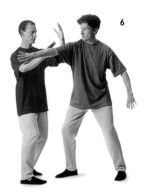

6

Working with a Partner

IN TAI CHI partnerwork two people interact in a cycle of pushing and yielding. Pushing hands offers a way of testing the solidity of movements learned in the solo form and it is a useful training technique for martial practice. Tai chi partner exercises also provide a safe, playful environment for experimenting with ways of dealing with other people. They offer possibilities for changing ingrained patterns of behavior and transforming the way one responds to situations in everyday life.

Quite early on in a tai chi course many teachers introduce their students to partnerwork This consists of taking turns at pushing a partner and reacting to their responses, and then being the one to receive and respond to the pushes. The apparent simplicity can be deceptive, however, because in partner practice, all the body structures and shapes learned in solo practice are applied.

Partnerwork follows a set of guiding principles, just as solo practice does. At the heart of these is natural way (see page 17). In partnerwork, natural way may be brought to life by learning to respond to the partner's movements rather than using force against force to dominate a situation, which has no permanent benefits. Tai chi teaches the wisdom of learning to respond to the needs of the moment.

However, while recognizing the importance of responding, tai chi also teaches the principle of remaining centered and grounded. This is known as holding one's space. Tai chi supports this process physically and emotionally through the structure and alignment of the body during a stance or movement.

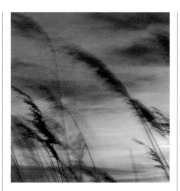

ABOVE *A reed in the wind is an inspiring embodiment of the qualities of tai chi natural way. With its roots embedded in the soil, it holds its space while responding to the varying pressures of the wind.*

Tai chi in no way a substitute for psychotherapy, but it does teach the art of dealing with emotions on a physical level. For example, partner practice encourages people to look honestly at themselves. The shape or position of the body and its effectiveness in dealing with a difficult situation, such as an incoming push, is a good indicator of a person's stance in life. In exchanges of pushing and yielding, receiving and giving, there are moments when patterns of over- or under-assertiveness become clear. Tai chi guides people toward achieving a balance.

Partnerwork also encourages the quality of acceptance. It is easy to suppress feelings and even experiences, and progress in tai chi depends on being able to pinpoint apprehension or anger, which manifest themselves visibly as extreme muscular tension. By recognizing such feelings the energy of fear can be transformed into courage and the energy of anger might be borrowed to bring clarification.

THE PROCESSES

The processes of listening and receiving, choosing, and giving, described on the opposite page, are applied by employing four simple techniques. The first is touch, the basic medium for contact and communication between two people. Sticking, the second technique, narrows the scope of touch by focusing it on a small area. The area of contact between two people becomes a channel for information to pass through. Joining happens when partners allow their feelings to extend into and envelop each other. Following is the fourth technique, and it involves carefully listening to and observing another person, and responding to their movements.

THE PROCESSES

In any tai chi partner exchange a clear sequence of events takes place as a recurring cycle, always in the same order: listening; receiving; choosing; giving. Think about how you use each of these qualities in your life. Can you find ways of incorporating a quality that feels uncomfortable?

1 Listening

This quality is at the hub of partner interaction and is carefully developed in tai chi. As if taking part in a conversation, you learn to listen through touch to the qualities (such as strength and direction) of your partner's push. As well as physical contact, the practice demands heightened sensitivity and awareness, so that you tune into your partner's intention.

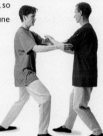

2 Receiving

This is a deep-seated yin or feminine quality (which men need to develop as much as women). Being able to receive incoming energy enables you to neutralize it. The depth of this quality needs to match the incoming energy's force, direction, and power.

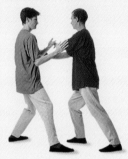

3 Choosing

By holding the space and surrendering to the force of the incoming push, the receiving partner has neutralized the threat and reaches a position of choice. From here the receiver can disengage; the partners can stay in contact but do nothing; or they can complete a cycle and the receiving partner clearly gives or directs the finished push back toward the other person.

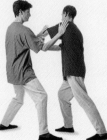

4 Giving/directing

This is a yang or masculine quality (which women need to develop as well as men). It is an energy that moves out, away from you in a clear direction, to wherever you choose to send it. It complements and balances the force of the incoming energy.

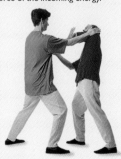

PUSHING HANDS

The techniques of touch, stick, join, follow, listen, receive, choose, and give combine in Pushing Hands to make total response possible in relating to another person.

Sticking

This is a two-person exercise, and you need to find a place to practice with enough space to move around. Begin by standing side by side. Carry out the exercise twice, for one to two minutes at a time, first with your eyes open, then with them closed, then change roles.

PARTNER A

Rest your right palm lightly on your partner's left wrist, and when the wrist begins to move, follow it, trying to maintain the same light pressure with your palm. Wherever the wrist leads, your palm must follow.

PARTNER B

From the moment the palm of your partner's hand touches your wrist, begin to move your forearm freely but at a steady pace, and keep moving it throughout. Do not stop moving or try to escape your partner's palm.

A Fighting Art

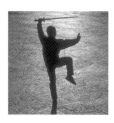

ABOVE *Every tai chi posture has a martial application, and the body makes the same graceful shapes in the martial applications of the art.*

FOR MUCH OF *its long history tai chi has been a respected fighting art. Its martial forms are thought to have evolved centuries ago from "external" or "hard" arts – rather like today's karate or kung fu – into an "internal" art, founded on inner strength and concentration. The change is said to have been made by the legendary Taoist sage Chang San-feng, who, it is related, saw a fight between a snake and a bird. Struck by the ability of snake and bird to yield, so that neither could overcome the other, Chang modified his hard fighting art to a "softer" one, in which attack might come from withdrawal, and defense might be based on neutralizing blows instead of using hard force.*

Students often branch out into martial applications as a way of adding an extra dimension to tai chi practice. In fact, everyone could benefit from seeing how each posture can be adapted to a martial situation. It clarifies the intention behind the postures and it brings focus to their practice.

Tai chi strikes a balance between the expression of yang or masculine aggression and the development of the yin quality of inner softness. All tai chi students – women and men – need to learn to express yang energy. Tai chi is not an evasive martial art – it is as aggressive as it needs to be. There is no mistaking the impact of a forceful punch.

Everyone who studies tai chi also needs to understand how to neutralize or absorb an incoming force, when and how to give way in order to conserve energy, and how the hidden face of yielding is attack. Cultivating the true martial spirit is as much about self-development as it is about self-defense.

A PAIR FORM

The principles of partner practice are the basis of tai chi as a fighting art, so understanding Pushing Hands is central to the sequences illustrated here, which are typical of the stages through which you might be taught the martial form.

Partner exercises train you to be fully present. They dissolve anticipation, teaching you to focus on what is happening and deal with it, rather than imagine what might happen. Pushing Hands in martial arts practice involves learning many different partner exercises. Some are choreographed, some improvised, and there are others with fixed and moving steps. Through them you learn theoretical responses to imagined situations. Once you have learned the basic moves in Single and Double Pushing Hands (right), you can begin to improvise. Free Pushing trains you to understand when different techniques are most appropriate.

Single pushing hands

This exercise develops basic listening, sticking, and yielding skills, and is often used as an introduction to partner exercises. You and your partner stand facing each other in a bow and arrow stance with the palm and wrist of your left or right hand in contact. You alternately push and receive in a continuous cycle.

Double pushing hands

This extension of Single Pushing Hands, using both hands instead of just one, offers more possibilities. The illustration shows part of the Wardoff, Rollback, Press, and Push sequence of Pushing Hands.

Free pushing

Students familiar with the basic principles of yielding and neutralizing in partnerwork are then given the opportunity to try free pushing – when you do not know whether your partner will push or yield. Free pushing makes it possible to apply any of the eight basic postures and respond more spontaneously.

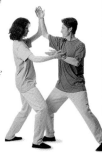

Da Lu ("big rollback")

This choreographed movement is first learned as a solo form, then put together with a partner. It develops the ability to step and move while applying hand techniques. There are many forms of Da Lu; the one shown here is common in Cheng Man-ch'ing style.

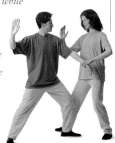

San Shou

The San Shou is what is known as a fast form. It is usually taught to students only after three years' practice. It is learned as two solo forms, two sides to a choreographed piece for two players. As a solo practice, the speed at which it runs highlights the many circles, spirals, and centrifugal forces not so easily felt in ordinary form.

TAI CHI WEAPONS FORMS

In tai chi practice today the sword and spear are employed as a means of improving agility and alertness, and never in combat. Learning to use tai chi weapons raises the body's energy levels and channels the energy outward, heightening coordination, focus, balance, and mental alertness.

The long sword

In China the long sword is known as the weapon of the scholar and the gentleman. The long sword is said to have been used as a tool by Taoist sages and is ascribed with magical powers. It is generally considered the hardest weapon to learn, requiring swiftness, deft footwork, flexibility, and sharpness of spirit.

The broad sword

The broad sword is a slashing weapon that uses large, circular, sweeping movements, generating considerable force from a relaxed center. It is a good weapon for practice, as it mobilizes both the spine and the torso.

The spear

The movements of the spear are strong, linear, well-extended thrusts joined with deflections. These yang movements develop clarity and decisiveness.

The staff

The staff is commonly associated with hard external fighting forms developed in China in the 600s. Yet the principles of tai chi can be put into practice with a staff, just as with a sword or spear.

Camouflaged weapons

In ancient China, objects of daily use, such as canes and fans, could double as practical aids to self-defense.

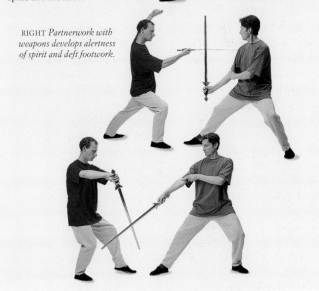

RIGHT *Partnerwork with weapons develops alertness of spirit and deft footwork.*

Cultivating Energy

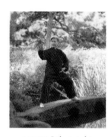

QIGUNG (OR CHI KUNG) *is an approach to exercise that complements tai chi. In fact the two are so closely related that some teachers practice what they call "tai chi qigung." Posture, movement, breathing, visualization, meditation, and focus are central to both, and both are health-giving exercises. But whereas tai chi emphasizes partner practice and has martial applications, qigung is largely a solo practice with less emphasis on interaction with others. Qigung means "energy work" and, essentially, it focuses on cultivating chi or life energy to promote well-being and vitality. Like tai chi, however, qigung encourages self-development.*

ABOVE *Like tai chi, qigung is good to practice in a clear, clean, and bright environment, either in or out of doors.*

Because tai chi and qigung are so similar, they are often confused. Qigung is commonly defined as exercises for health, and tai chi is sometimes explained as movements for fighting. Both definitions are limited, since tai chi is also a healing art and qigung can teach how to conserve and focus energy in martial training. By contrast with the flow of movement of tai chi, qigung tends to be more static. Internally, however, it seeks to build and move energy. Tai chi, by contrast, draws energy from the body and directs it outward through pushing hands and weapons forms.

Qigung and tai chi have evolved from common origins now buried deep in antiquity. Through the ages qigung has developed into many different styles and approaches. For example, neigung is called the art of internal power because its emphasis is on developing the body's internal energy through exercises, postures, breathing, and visualization. It was once called upon to harden the body

for battle by training it to tolerate blows. Adepts described how training began by gently striking the body's vital points with a small bag of Chinese beans, and progressed to blows of increasing force with larger and heavier implements. Today, neigung is used to strengthen confidence in pushing hands or fighting practice, and to deepen relaxation.

Tai chi and qigung complement each other perfectly and are often taught together. Qigung exercises are often used to prepare for the tai chi form (see pages 62–115). Tai chi qigung exploits the similarities between the two to develop energy-building techniques. For example, a tai chi posture might be held for five minutes to build energy, or treated as a solo exercise and repeated many times to work the muscles and speed the circulation of the blood.

Many different types of qigung are practiced today. Indeed, this book has taken a quigung approach to its presentation of the tai chi form. Many quigung exercises are

aimed at directing the mind and the life force to the organs, the joints, and other parts of the body to promote health. Opposite is a short qigung sequence that can be practiced on its own or can be used as a preparation for the tai chi form.

CENTERING

Begin each exercise standing with your weight distributed evenly and your feet one shoulder width apart. Spend a few minutes softening and opening each reference point (see page 45).

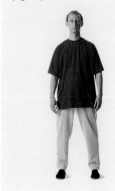

A QIGUNG SEQUENCE

This short qigung sequence can be practiced on its own or added to the preparation exercises on pages 58–61. Start each exercise by centering (see left). The exercises will relax you, stimulate circulation, release unwanted energy, and leave you feeling refreshed and tranquil.

EARTH BREATHING

This exercise relaxes and the working of the legs and arms stimulates circulation. Imagine yourself breathing the earth inward, filling your body from toes to crown. Tune into the rhythm of your breath, imagining it activating and clearing the energy centers. The out-breath releases unwanted energy and returns you to the earth.

1 Bring all your weight onto your right leg, and sit deeply into it. Slide your left foot forward, lifting the heel slightly.

2 Feel connected to the earth. Breathe in deeply, and as you do so, slowly rise by straightening your right leg, and let your arms float up.

3 Breathe out naturally while sitting your weight deeply into your right leg and lowering your hands to the lower tantien.

4 Repeat steps 1–3 at least two more times before transferring your weight to the left leg and repeating them three times on the left side.

5 Transfer your weight back to the right leg and repeat the cycle on the right side, bringing your arms out to the sides and raising and lowering them in step 2 in the manner of slow-motion flying. Repeat the cycle once more on the left leg. Finish by centering.

SUNRISE

This exercise lightens and refreshes the spirit.

1 Sit deeply into both feet and very slowly raise your hands to chest level, imagining that you lift the sun from under the earth up through your feet.

2 Imagine the sun fills your heart and that its light fills your whole body and bursts out to shine in the space around you. Raise your hands and your face toward the sky.

3 Relax your face and turn forward, and, lowering your arms, open them fully so they extend upward and outward. Enjoy this position of radiance.

4 Finish by centering, then repeat steps 1–3 twice.

SUNSET

This position leaves you feeling quiet, contained, and peaceful. Its gathering and calming moves complement the upward and outward energy of Sunrise, above.

1 Circle your arms upward in a large arc, finishing with your fingertips about 2 inches apart opposite your face. Respond with a sense of gathering.

2 Move your hands slowly and gracefully down to rest by your sides like the sun setting.

3 Repeat steps 1 and 2 two more times, then rest your hands on the lower tantien. Imagine all your energy centers alive and balanced.

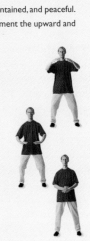

Tai Chi for Life

TO MOVE WITH *grace, power, and beauty, to harmonize with the heartbeat, the breath, and the cosmos is to receive the greatest gifts tai chi can offer. Yet practicing the movements can take as little as ten minutes, so what about the rest of the day? Tai chi is not an art that need be restricted to "training," or imprisoned in a time slot. It should never become a treadmill activity that dulls the imagination. It is a creative activity which, allowed to extend beyond practice into everyday life, will invigorate the mind and enrich the spirit. To cultivate this aspect of tai chi is to open a channel through which one's buried creative urges can surface.*

LEFT *Spontaneity is as essential to tai chi practice as it is to a child's play.*

Beginners often ask how much they need to practice. At the beginning it is a good idea to aim at practicing for about 10 minutes a day. For steady improvement it is important to practice regularly. However, it is equally necessary to have the right approach to discipline. To force oneself to practice is to adopt a rigid, over zealous approach, and although commitment is essential, so is inspiration. Practice must be based on intuition, feeling, and common sense. To be fruitful tai chi needs to be practiced with passion.

Tai chi embodies the Taoist principles, and the idea behind practice is to bring these to life. They are simple: tai chi expresses the polarity of opposites – yin and yang, open and closed, full and empty, and central balance and the dynamic equilibrium between them.

One way of keeping practice alive is to make one pair of polarities or one quality the theme of the day or the week, observing it at work when practicing the simplest movements, and noticing how one quality, such as listening, feels in relation to its opposite. It is easy to extend the idea of exploring a quality beyond practice by observing different aspects of it as they occur in daily life, noticing one's own habits of listening or failing to listen during interactions with other people, and

KITCHEN PRACTICE

Extend practice time by always having a couple of possibilities up your sleeve. Perhaps you want to develop a stepping technique or get a better sense of how your spine turns. Then, those endless minutes when coffee is warming or bread toasting stand out as ideal times for practice. In a slow line at a checkout, practice feeling weight transfer from one foot to the other. In your car in a traffic gridlock, breathe more deeply, become centered, massage your hands. Any time you find yourself waiting, think of it as another opportunity for practice.

observing how and when they listen. Eventually it becomes second nature to explore the qualities in daily life, noticing links between their appearance in different situations and in tai chi movements. Exercises of this kind can sharpen the awareness.

Nevertheless, learning the form does mean attending regular, disciplined practice sessions for as long as a year, and it is important during this time not to lose sight of personal needs. The mind and body are constantly changing. One day there may be a need for grounding, and another may bring a need to move faster, or to direct the attention outward. This is where free practice and freestyle movement (see pages 128–29) are most valuable.

To acknowledge tai chi as a practice that affects the health of body, mind, and soul is to open to the broad range of experiences it offers. Exercising is only one aspect of practice. Some of its many avenues are explored in the following pages.

CREATIVITY AND EXPRESSION

Creativity springs from the urge to express. It begins with the natural outward expression of inner feelings, and from there often springs a desire to communicate emotion in singing or playing music, or in poetry. Children are naturally uninhibited, but as they mature, they learn to suppress certain feelings. It is now well understood that in the more Northern cultures generally, emotions tend to be more repressed than in Southern areas, and that in certain north European societies especially, men find it difficult to address their feelings.

To inhibit one's natural expression creates stress, and in extreme cases stress replaces expression. When the body is stressed, tension builds in the muscles in response to a perceived danger: the fight or flight mechanism. Hormones, such as adrenaline, are released, which raise the blood pressure, speed up the heart, and increase the breathing rate. When the situation calls for physical action, such as fleeing, this energy is utilized, and the hormone production subsides, but when the danger takes the form of a frightening bank statement or a crisis in a relationship, the gathered energy remains unused and the hormones continue to circulate. Hormones may build up in the bloodstream, and chronic stress may lead to illnesses as serious as stroke, heart disease, and perhaps even cancer.

Tai chi works at all levels to prevent the build up of tension, break the stress cycle, relieve symptoms, and so prevent illness from developing. It generates energy in the hui yin and lower tantien energy centers (see pages 40–41), which rises as part of a cycle that moves to the top of the head and down to the pelvis. This energy tries to find an outlet, and people often feel stifled in the throat and chest if they deny the powerful and natural urge to express it, perhaps through an outlet for creativity. Tai chi also has a massaging effect on mind and body, so it works against the build up of chronic tension. After practice, sitting or lying down to rest and waiting in a receptive way may bring the root cause of tension to the surface. Once it has become apparent, it can be dealt with.

Creative expression is one way of utilizing the energy generated by tai chi and people often discover a heartfelt need to continue with the drawing they abandoned years ago, or to buy a new camera, to join a choir, or audition for a part in a play. There are many different forms of expression. One person might decide to have a child; another to travel for a while. Before you find the right form of self-expression, you may experience uncertainty and confusion, or physical symptoms of frustration. Bear in mind that speaking is one of the simplest, most accessible, and natural forms of self-expression. Begin by listening to your own voice.

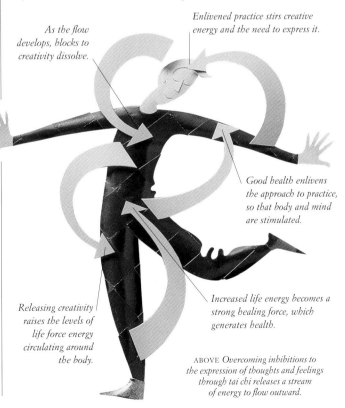

As the flow develops, blocks to creativity dissolve.

Enlivened practice stirs creative energy and the need to express it.

Good health enlivens the approach to practice, so that body and mind are stimulated.

Releasing creativity raises the levels of life force energy circulating around the body.

Increased life energy becomes a strong healing force, which generates health.

ABOVE *Overcoming inhibitions to the expression of thoughts and feelings through tai chi releases a stream of energy to flow outward.*

Nature and the Elements

IN TRADITIONAL CHINESE *philosophy the five elements – water, wood, fire, metal, and earth – are thought of as the basis of all life on earth, and for hundreds of years Western philosophy saw the universe as composed of earth, water, fire, and air. Even without the guidance of philosophy it is easy to see how these elements are the raw materials of nature. Tai chi is a system of movement that follows the natural way of things, so practicing tai chi must involve learning about nature and about ourselves, for the self is a fundamental part of nature. The study of tai chi is an investigation into the very essence of life.*

Everyone seems to have an unconscious familiarity and sense of ease with one or perhaps two of the elements. Many people, for example, would agree that a solid, thickset, steady person could be said to be earthy, and a lightly built person is more like air or fire. Our language is full of expressions that derive from the ancient concept of the elements. People with a vivid imagination are often described as air-headed, and we talk of fiery tempers. Each of the four elements has its distinctive characteristics.

The objective of working with the elements is to widen the understanding of their qualities beyond what is familiar, to recognize your own elemental qualities, and to encourage people to experience working with the elements in many different ways. A naturally earthy person can experience how it feels to be light, and a light person can discover the solid nature of earth as a real physical experience. This exploration of elemental qualities can be exciting. It is like adding more pieces to the jigsaw of personal life. It extends the breadth and quality of individual

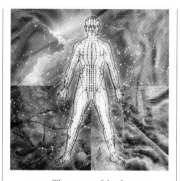

ABOVE *The concept of the elements is central to all Chinese healing arts, including acupuncture and moxibustion, and Chinese herbal medicine.*

experience and adds new possibilities to the range of responses you can bring to daily encounters with nature and other people.

You can, as the exercises shown on these pages demonstrate, draw inspiration from nature, from cities, built up areas, or cultivated county-side. The fruits of every investigation into the elements can then be brought back into the tai chi form. Discovering how it feels to move in a light, airy way, a solid, earthy way, a flowing watery way, or an energetic, fiery way enhances practice and makes it more enjoyable.

INSPIRATION FROM NATURE

Pictures and records show that all through human history people have sought to fulfil a need for communication with nature. The Taoists are remembered today more for their study of nature than for other aspects of their philosophy.

To draw inspiration from nature is to experience something of the essence of life. The following exercises explore different ways of communing with nature.

1 *Go to a wild place where the elements seem raw and clear. You may know a river you can go to sit beside, or a hillside or an outcrop of rock you can lie on. Wild places are no longer plentiful, so you may need to plan this exercise as if it were a pilgrimage of a day or longer. Go camping somewhere you can light a camp fire, take a trip to a wild area of coast.*

2 *When you arrive, swim in the river or the sea, feel the wind and rain on your skin, watch the clouds. Look and listen, absorbing the teachings of nature. Understand how nature works. Notice the interaction between all the elements in creating life.*

DISCOVERING THE ELEMENTS

The elements are everywhere, and in these exercises you learn to recognize them and to embody their qualities in movement. This is a creative and rewarding process because it uses the power of the imagination to create tangible effects. The qualities of the elements can be embodied through the tai chi postures or in free movement (see pages 128–29). The following exercise shows you how to do this through visualization.

Visualization

The aim of the visualizations is to enable you to implement the energy of the different elements. During visualization you should sit, stand, or lie down, as you feel appropriate. Search your imagination for an image related to the subject, allowing time to find the image that exactly expresses your feelings or needs of the moment. When visualizing fire, for instance, you might imagine a cosy log fire, or a furnace. Once you have found an appropriate image, examine it closely until you can almost feel it. Imagine its essence penetrating the cells of your body so you become part of it. Spend all the time you need to incorporate the image into your body. Afterward, notice what difference it has made as you move in tai chi or go about your daily business.

ELEMENT: EARTH
Associated qualities: Rootedness, steadiness, groundedness, solidity, strength, stability.
Visualization: Call to mind anything earthy – a mountain, freshly tilled soil, an animal such as an elephant or a Shire horse.

ELEMENT: WATER
Associated qualities: Relaxation, power, knowing your place, ease, effortlessness, no wasting of energy, tirelessness, flow, movement, fearlessness, simplicity, change.
Visualization: This may be anything from a lake to a raindrop, from the calm sea to a raging torrent.

ELEMENT: FIRE
Associated qualities: Energy, warmth, light, joy, comfort, speed, cleansing, transformation, decisiveness.
Visualization: This may be sunshine, the glowing embers of a camp fire, or lightning.

ELEMENT: AIR
Associated qualities: Lightness, sensitivity, feeling, alertness, communicability, clarity, swift change.
Visualization: Think of the different aspects of air, from soft, warm, scented night air to a harsh, cold, wintry blast.

ELEMENTS IN URBAN LIFE

The elements are all around – in cities and in cultivated countryside. Notice how the water behaves when you are bathing or showering. Stand by an open window and feel the air with your hands, on your face, and when you breathe. Stand outdoors and face the sunshine, closing your eyes and feeling its warmth and light. At any moment of any day it is possible to awaken your life with elemental awareness.

CREATING A SPECIAL PLACE

Create a special place in your home for a collection of objects symbolic of the elements. A rock you came across one day, a feather, a bowl of water just from the faucet, and a candle can create a strongly elemental and beautiful atmosphere to keep you in contact with nature.

CAUTION

Light fires only where they will do no harm, and make certain they are completely extinguished when you leave. Swim only where it is safe, and never alone. Stand in the wind only where you are not in danger.

BELOW *A candle lit in your home can create a special place, where you can feel in touch with the elements.*

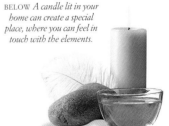

Freestyle Movement

EVERYONE KNOWS HOW *to move, but few adults are aware that, as they have matured, the range of movements of which they are capable has steadily decreased. Moreover, many people's movements are restricted to a narrow band of activity – sitting on a chair, lying, standing to work at tasks, walking – and they have forgotten altogether how to move freely,. Freestyle movement loosens up the body and dissolves inhibitions, bringing deeper understanding and increased vitality to the more disciplined movements of the tai chi form.*

Although at first it might seem easy to move without the restrictions of form, it can be hard to know where to begin. A good starting point is to remember the Taoist principles of tai chi. Freestyle movement might equally be termed Radical Taoist Movement, because it is based on the seven basic qualities of yin and yang, open and closed, full and empty, and central equilibrium. It develops these polarities as human qualities, exploring them in movement.

In recent years a fashion has emerged for aerobic activities and working out on machines in gyms, indicating an awareness of the need to widen the body's regular range of movements. But that type of training tends to exercise just one physical aspect of the body. Tai chi treats body and mind as a single unit, and the exercises on these pages are designed to stimulate the body to restore free, holistic movement. These introductory exercises are guidelines to

enable people to enjoy movement for movement's sake. Real power develops when the beginner abandons the core exercises and begins to improvise and explore.

It is important to take regular notice of what freestyle movement contributes to formal tai chi practice. It means moving according to the principles at the hub of Taoist thinking and at the core of tai chi, and its effect is to bring meaning to the postures and empower the individual to move more exactly.

1 *Move into an open shape, then into a closed shape, taking careful notice of how different the two polarities feel. Repeat these movements, but this time, as you perform an open movement try to feel a little more open; and as you move into a closed position try to close yourself a little further. Notice the polarity increasing and the dynamic energy growing. Repeat the moves several times, always trying to take each polarity a little further.*

2 *Now add a second set of polarities, large and small, say. Try to define what happens. Explore different combinations: large and open; large and closed; small and open; small and closed. Then add another polarity. Continue this exploration until you feel like finishing, then continue with new polarities in another session.*

RADICAL TAOIST MOVEMENT

Before you begin to move, pause and focus on one of the polarities. Open and closed is used as an example here, but you could choose light and heavy, fast and slow; awareness directed outward, awareness directed inward; or any other pair of polarities. Follow the guidelines below, and you will soon begin to move in a way that is alive, real, and fun. This is exploring radical Taoist movement, journeying through a landscape of experiences, some of which feel familiar and comfortable, others strange and rather disturbing. Expect occasionally to feel surprisingly comfortable with an unfamiliar movement.

Lying and rolling

Lie in a clean, comfortable place where you can let yourself relax completely. Spend as much time as you feel you want to in this wonderful, restorative position. When you are ready, roll over and, if you feel you want to, roll over the ground. Rest after moving if you feel you need to. While lying and while rolling, think about how it feels to have your body close to the earth.

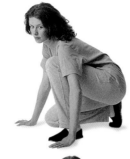

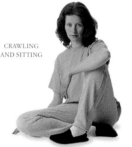

CRAWLING
AND SITTING

Crawling and sitting

Lie on your back and lift your head and then your shoulders and trunk until you are in a sitting position. You will notice that you need to exert a great deal of muscular effort and tension to do this. Now lie on your back again, and this time roll over to the left while drawing in your right knee and you will find yourself in a crawling position almost without effort. Spend some time crawling, then experiment with lowering your hips until you find a sitting position. Practice this exercise a number of times, easing your way as effortlessly as you can between lying and crawling and sitting. While you do so, notice what use you make of your arms and hips. Think about how it feels to roll and crawl and sit. Does it bring any memories into mind?

Ease of movement

Your body moves on three levels: the horizontal – lying or perhaps rolling; the semi-upright – crawling, sitting, perhaps crouching or squatting;

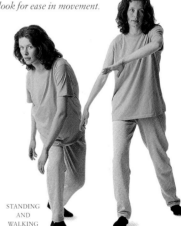

LYING AND
ROLLING

and the vertical – standing, walking, running, and so on. These movements reflect the evolution of human mobility from infant to adult, and the exercises take you progressively from the first to the last, exploring the potential for movement of each stage. Work on a pattern of moving and resting, and occasionally stretching out. Breathe deeply and do not hold your breath when moving. Let your breathing complement your body shapes and movements. When you feel at ease with these movements, try exploring themes and launching into new experiences. Run through the basic sequence and then improvise, letting the practice unfold.

Standing and walking

Whenever you move between the three basic levels, think of moving with ease and fluidity, not in straight lines but in circles and spirals. When you are ready, spiral your way from sitting into a standing position, then back to a sitting position. Repeat this movement many times until you feel comfortable with it. Then, perhaps on a different occasion, experiment with walking and other types of vertical movement: skipping, hopping, jumping, running, and combinations of these. Always look for ease in movement.

STANDING
AND
WALKING

Tai Chi at Work

PEOPLE THESE DAYS *lead very busy lives and have little time to spare for interests such as tai chi. It is worthwhile, however, finding a way of fitting a class and practice time into a weekly schedule, however packed it may be. Learning to be flexible is an important part of a holistic approach to health. Tai chi is an investment that will pay dividends in a calmer outlook, improved concentration, and a feeling of greater control over the events of the day. Better time management begins with making time for daily practice.*

Before making any plans to start practicing tai chi it is essential to be convinced that it will be worth all the effort. The decision must not spring from a sense of duty ("I ought to get more exercise;" or "I really ought to do it for my health") but from a yearning to give something to yourself, from an inner desire to learn tai chi. Practice must be something every learner looks forward to. It must never be enforced, never an activity that has to be stuck to because you have made a promise to yourself.

The health benefits of long-term practice have been explained. In addition, tai chi shows people ways of dealing with the tensions of working life, and how to maintain an equilibrium so that concentration, relationships both at work and outside it, do not suffer, and well-being is maintained.

LEFT *Partnerwork and pushing hands explore relationships and enable you to develop new ways of dealing with people.*

A real desire to learn tai chi comes from deep inside, from self-love, a form of energy responsible for the well being of body, mind, heart, and soul. If you are really motivated, your commitment will work out because it is based on inspiration and not on discipline.

A PRACTICAL APPROACH TO EXERCISE

EXERCISE	DURATION	FIND IT ON
Turning	1 minute	*page 58*
Rainbow Circle	2 minutes	*page 58*
Snake Shake your whole body from top to toe, including hands and fingers	30 seconds	*page 61*
Push as a Key Move posture in a repeating cycle of back, down, and forward	2 minutes	*page 57*
Massage your hands	30 seconds	*page 13*
Massage your face	30 seconds	*page 13*
Massage your ears	30 seconds	*page 13*
Beginning posture	2 minutes	*page 64*
Ward off left, Ward off right, Rollback, Press, Push, and Single Whip	2 minutes	*page 66–70*
TOTAL TIME	11 minutes	

Tai Chi at Leisure

TAI CHI IS *the main recreation of many people, but for an increasing number it is being taken up as a valuable supplement to a major sport, such as golf or basketball. Tai chi exercises the whole body, emphasizes posture, balance, and energy management, and it develops body awareness and mental alertness, and these qualities are in high demand for greater enjoyment and success in a number of other activities. This page shows how tai chi can be the perfect backup to improving performance in sports ranging from horse riding to soccer, but it can be equally valuable in increasing success in more sedentary interests, from poker to pool to playing the guitar.*

LEFT *The quality of a golf swing may improve as a result of improved concentration and better coordination developed during tai chi practice.*

It is now a truism that a comfortably relaxed body works better, and it follows that relaxing will improve performance in almost any activity, physical or mental. Tai chi teaches how to dispel tension and control energy flow, and these qualities are now being used by professionals in a number of sports to improve concentration and the ability to relax during moments of great tension.

Every aspect of tai chi can be useful preparation for other physical activities. The preparatory exercises, for example (see pages 58–61), are an excellent way of warming up. Tai chi works better than many standard warm-up exercises practiced before different sports, in that it prepares the mind as well as conditioning the body. The static exercises provide a transition between preparation and performance, clearing mental space as if preparing the mind for action. The exercises have a grounding effect, which brings the player into the heart of the moment, improving the ability to focus.

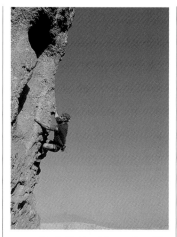

ABOVE *Rock-climbing defies gravity, while tai chi keeps the feet firmly planted on the ground, yet there are common links.*

TEAM SPORTS

Gathering energy inward and channeling it to wherever it is needed is fundamental to tai chi. Learning how to manage and conserve energy through tai chi practice increases stamina, improves teamwork, and so enhances quality playing time in team sports and games, such as baseball, soccer, and basketball.

ROCK-CLIMBING

Success in rock-climbing is linked directly to the ability to relax in difficult situations. This is studied closely in pushing hands. Climbers who also practice tai chi report that their balance and ease of movement is improved.

HORSE RIDING

Riders have noticed that tai chi raises their body awareness, so that they are able to center through the horse. Partner training in tai chi naturally heightens a rider's awareness of the relationship with the horse. The qualities of listening and sticking, important in tai chi, are experienced through contact with the horse's mouth through the reins, as well as through the sitting posture.

GOLF

Better coordination is one of the effects of tai chi. Success in golf relies on excellent coordination to make a perfect swing, so tai chi can improve one's handicap!

Achieving Self-Fulfillment

MANY BEGINNERS ENJOY *the wonderfully relaxed way they feel after tai chi practice. As they progress, however, some encounter difficulties with physical aspects of tai chi, such as balance, emotional restrictions, or resistance to working with a partner. Challenging these impediments is the essence of the art; beginning tai chi means setting out on a journey toward greater self-fulfillment and deeper relationships with others.*

LEFT *One of the aims of tai chi is to restore to the adult body the flexibility it enjoyed in infancy.*

Tai chi cultivates ease of movement, something modern lifestyle inhibits. We sit on chairs and are carried by escalators. We can almost get away without moving. One of the aims of tai chi is to restore some of the wonderful flexibility of movement children naturally have. Adults, by contrast, need to work at loosening up. Practicing journeying from lying on the floor to sitting and then to standing, in a smooth, gradual, unbroken sequence of movements is a good way of overcoming resistance to movement. Another is to squat for a minute or two now and again. Squatting opens the ankle joints, stretches the Achilles, tendons, and mobilizes the hip joints.

Emotional blocks sometimes prevent us from moving freely. Western men have tended to be especially inhibited. Although society is changing rapidly, men still tend to be competitive and overaggressive, or to have lost their sense of warrior spirit. Modern men are more open to a different type of strength based on intelligence and flexibility. Tai chi shows them how to redress the imbalances caused by overcompensation, find a balance, and become a new kind of "gentle man." Women, on the other hand, rarely know their own strength. They are simply not in touch with it. Many are afraid to find it, and if they discover it, they are shocked. By developing their awareness, tai chi can show women that they also have warrior energy. Practicing the punch is one way of

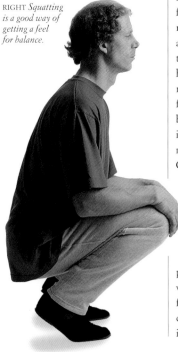

RIGHT *Squatting is a good way of getting a feel for balance.*

doing this. Just making a fist and considering how it feels can bring to the surface a process that is going on beneath.

Tai chi is an exacting discipline. Executing several complex movements simultaneously demands perfect concentration. Learners are sometimes surprised to encounter an internal resistance to learning the form that may manifest itself by repeating the same mistake over and again. One way of overcoming this is to take notes in class and practice at home; another is to visualize the resistance as a bung, stopping the flow of life energy like a cork stops bubbles escaping from a bottle. It is also important to check one's motivation for taking up tai chi. Giving into urging from strong-minded friends who know what is best can leave people in an unconscious state of resentment that can surface as some form of resistance or mental block.

The following pages present the personal accounts of some people who practice tai chi today. Their different stories all show that, when it comes to tai chi, personal motivation is paramount.

Growing and Changing

STIFF-LIMBED, INFLEXIBLE-minded adult tai-chi learners have to work at regaining some of the softness and flexibility of their childhood bodies, and their youthful spontaneity. Children play unaffectedly, express their emotions uninhibitedly, and indulge their natural creativity unselfconsciously. Why, then, would they need tai chi? Change – a key theme of childhood – may be part of the answer. Physically, mentally, and emotionally children grow up with change as a part of their everyday experience. Tai chi movements can give them an inner stability.

Tai chi can provide a way of channeling children's natural enthusiasm for play. Based as it is on the concept of yin-yang or polarity of opposites, tai chi offers endless possibilities for exploring movement. Children have fun investigating the movement potential of concepts such as large and small, loud and quiet, round and sharp, light and heavy. Most are in touch with the imagination and able to access qualities in their bodies through visualization.

Tai chi seems to benefit children around the age of eight especially. It appears to help them establish a solidity and develop a sense of self. Children of that age group still love to act out being wild, ferocious, or still, but they are beginning to want to try some of the postures from the form and wrangle with the structure and discipline that goes with them. When taught a short sequence they respond well to a chance to express their creativity.

During the often dramatic teen years tai chi can act as an anchor, enabling young people to retain a solid sense of self while beginning to venture outward into the world and into new relations with other people. Through Pushing Hands teenagers can channel their physical energy, developing a familiarity with touch. Thinking about the principles underlying the practice can give

BELOW *The energy and creativity of children can be channeled into an exploration of tai chi movements.*

them an angle on the often confusing realms of interaction with other people, and a philosophy for dealing with them.

HOLDING A STANCE

Children display much greater flexibility than adults and their bodies are softer. It is important not to strain young bones, joints, ligaments, tendons, and muscles. They are still growing right into their late teenage years. Whereas in adult tai chi the emphasis is often on holding a posture to develop stamina or build strength, children and teenagers must be carefully guided. It can put strain on a young body and to stress a body that is still growing can be damaging.

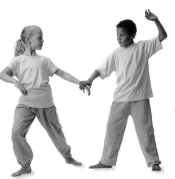
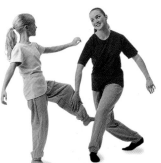
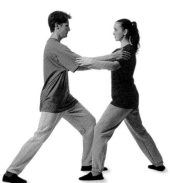

Tai Chi Experiences

THE FOLLOWING FOUR *pages present the stories of twelve people who have incorporated tai chi into their lives. They are people of varying ages and backgrounds. For some, their journey into tai chi began only recently, and for others, tai chi has been a regular part of their lives for years. What these diverse tai chi students have in common is that all have benefited from their practice of the art. Here, they explain the different ways in which tai chi has enriched their lives.*

Alison Ford
AGE: 21
Social worker
BEGAN TAI CHI: Six months ago

While she was taking her graduation examinations at college, Alison looked for something to ease the stress. Her mental tension was interwoven with emotional unease because she felt depressed. She wanted to slow down inside her head and find a sense of direction in her life. She was drawn to qigong, which helped but did not fully meet her needs.

After leaving college Alison took up tai chi. She tried out different teachers and knew immediately when she found the right one. Now she has a renewed enthusiasm for life, and brings a different approach to it. Tai chi, she feels, has brought about the change. Rather than worry and try to work things out in her head, she now feels her way with decisions, and this, she says, is because tai chi has awoken a new sensitivity in her body. Recently, the value of tai chi has been recognized by her superiors at work, who have sponsored a ten-week tai chi course for her to take place at work.

And tai chi has had another effect on her inner life. It has put Alison in touch with a need to express herself that she had never recognized. At first she experienced it as an uncomfortable physical sensation in her chest and throat whenever she practiced. Encouraged by her teacher, she is beginning to express herself through drawing, and rekindling her love of singing, discovering, in the process, an exciting new world.

Harry Goldstein
AGE: 67
Retired, former business manager
BEGAN TAI CHI: Two years ago

Wanting to maintain a good level of health and fitness, and able to spend more time on himself, Harry has been enjoying tai chi since he retired. It was the need for exercise that first brought him to a class, but he now values his new ability to relax in stressful situations. He has developed greater tolerance of others. He is more aware of himself in relation to those around him and finds it easier to respond positively. His reactions have sharpened up, he has noticed, and he is generally more alert mentally.

Harry is surprised to find himself less physically inhibited than he was before starting tai chi. He has noticed a change in his body's capacity to heal after injury. Knocks, bumps, and one fall in particular have cleared up more quickly than has been his experience in the past.

Sonny Freeman
AGE: 13
School student
BEGAN TAI CHI:
Six weeks ago

Carla Freeman
AGE: 47
Housewife, Sonny's mother
BEGAN TAI CHI:
Six weeks ago

Some time before Sonny and his mother Carla joined a weekly tai chi class, Sonny had been looking for something he could do to build up his confidence and self-esteem. At first, seeking to develop his personal power, he tried aikido, but he later realized it was not really giving him what he needed. He was attracted to tai chi and found a local class, but because it was an adults' class, he had to nudge his mother

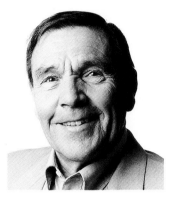

HARRY GOLDSTEIN

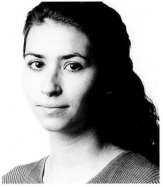

ALISON FORD

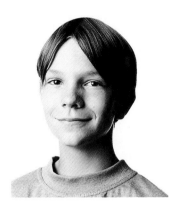

SONNY FREEMAN

into joining so he could accompany her. Sonny approached tai chi with realistic ideas of what he might achieve, he was not expecting tai chi to solve all his problems. He enjoys working on his own and likes to find things out for himself.

Sonny quickly discovered he was enjoying the non combative nature of tai chi. In aikido he was always picked on to be thrown because he was bigger than his classmates. After only six weeks he is feeling more relaxed, confident, and happier. He is not such a target at school and is handling the other guys better. He thinks some of them will come round to seeing things his way.

Carla is also realizing the benefits of tai chi. Her joints always used to hurt after the keep fit and aerobics classes she used to attend, but since she started tai chi, that has stopped. She is already experiencing higher energy levels, enjoying the exercise, and especially likes the manageable approach to meditation through earth breathing, sunrise and sunset, and other movements (see pages 122–123). She feels she can listen to people better now.

Donna Lopez

AGE: 33

Artist and art teacher

BEGAN TAI CHI: Nine years ago

A thesis she wrote during her final year at art school, in which she explored links between visionary art and Taoism, brought Donna in contact with tai chi. She was transfixed by the graceful movements and joined a class.

Soon after she began tai chi she found that only fifteen minutes' daily practice made her feel more relaxed physically while centering her mentally. This proved a great advantage, because she worked long hours into the night as a waitress to support her career as an artist. She went on to manage the restaurant and it was then that she realized how useful partnerwork can be. Through it she understood how she was relating to others, and was better able to build good relations with her staff and deal with customers' needs and demands. Through tai chi, she has learnt how to assert herself in a rewarding way, without dominating or being aggressive.

Practicing longer stances has strengthened her legs. Her spine and pelvis have freed up and tension in the muscles of her neck and shoulders has eased. Always keen on horse riding, she soon began to ride more lightly, to connect with the ground through her horse. She has also noticed that her balance has improved, and now finds horse riding altogether more satisfying.

Tai chi has become an important anchor during major life changes – through the breakup of her marriage and when she left her home and job. At difficult times like these, tai chi practice keeps energy levels high and maintains health. It earths the spirit. These strengths gave Donna the courage she needed to face the changes. Since these difficult times she has always used tai chi to enable her to live her life to the full.

Today, an artist and art teacher, she calls on the philosophies of tai chi to teach her how to let go and express herself more easily. She notices how people free up to paint and draw far more quickly and easily when they are involved in tai chi movement.

Maria Conti

AGE: 59
Cares for her mother
BEGAN TAI CHI: Eight years ago

Maria began practicing tai chi when she was 51, when she was suffering from stiffening ankles and lower back pain. Now she says she is stronger and more supple than when she was 30, and this has restored her confidence in her body, and renewed her sense of self-worth. When she began tai chi she was employed doing heavy kitchen work. Practice gave her the balance and coordination that enabled her to perform these tasks with greater ease than people 20 years her junior.

Over the years she has found that her health has improved, especially her resistance to infection, and her weight has stabilized. She is more relaxed, and she feels more balanced emotionally. She can see things much more clearly, and finds happiness in everyday events. Now Maria passes her inspiration onto others, running her own classes, including some for older people.

Roopi Patel

AGE: 33
Art student
BEGAN TAI CHI: Eight years ago

Roopi's study of tai chi was especially beneficial during her second pregnancy. She joined a class several of her friends were attending, just because it seemed fun. After about a year she signed up for a weekend workshop, which was to be a turning point in her life. The course focused on connecting with

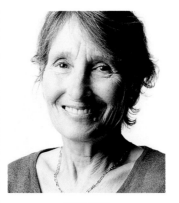

MARIA CONTI

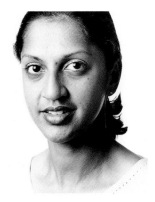

ROOPI PATEL

the pelvis, and it came at a time when Roopi was making a decision about whether to advance her career or have another child. Through tai chi she realized how much anxiety and fear she held in her pelvis from the difficult birth of her first child. The postures helped her achieve a feeling of freedom and empowerment as she met her fears. The experience restored her confidence in her body and gave her an emotional clarity. She realized that in fact she wanted to have another child.

For her pregnancy, Roopi drew up a health and fitness program, and used tai chi to make herself stick to it. She gave up cigarettes, and used tai chi postures to help her resist the urge to smoke. She was concerned that she might not be able to continue tai chi into the ninth month – would she have the flexibility and mobility? She should not have worried, she says. As she shed her inhibitions, she enjoyed being the star of the class – she felt an enjoyable satisfaction at wielding a sword when she had a huge, pregnant stomach. She went on to have a trouble-free home birth.

Cristina Neilsen

AGE: 70
Writer
BEGAN TAI CHI: 14 years ago

Cristina started tai chi when she was well into her fifties. She loved the flow of the movements and really enjoyed the learning process. When she began, she was worried about a pain that she thought might be the beginning of arthritis in her left knee. After a few months of careful guidance and regular practice, it had gone. Now, all signs of arthritis have disappeared. Cristina speaks of how her energy has increased with her age. She can now walk uphill easily, and she breathes better. She finds the discipline of the moves has improved her concentration and continues to maintain her mental alertness. At the same time, studying tai chi movement has given her an inner joy in free movement outside the form. It makes her more spontaneous and puts her in touch with a natural wildness in her spirit. She describes herself as a healthier and happier person than before she began tai chi.

Gerald Dupuis
AGE: 17
Studying for the international baccalaureate
BEGAN TAI CHI: Six weeks ago

Gerald has never been attracted to team and other sports, but he felt he needed exercise, and was looking for a form of physical recreation that would make him feel good when, shortly after leaving school, he came across tai chi.

He is enjoying his first experience of tai chi immensely, and is attracted by its non-competitive nature. The way of tai chi is already unfolding for him in exciting ways. For example, he is experiencing new physical sensations in his feet, and is enthusiastically exploring this new territory. Gerald looks upon his class as quality time for himself, a space in his life where he is free from the stresses of college and studies.

Raisa Malinski
AGE: 39
Company administrator
BEGAN TAI CHI: Five years ago

Having heard people talk about tai chi and seen a little of it here and there, Raisa eventually took it up. Over the last five years it has become an important part of her life. She has noticed marked changes slowly taking place in her physical condition. She has noticed marked improvements in her balance and coordination, she is more supple, and her circulation is better. She has a longer back than normal, which has caused outbreaks of back pain and she is regularly treated by an

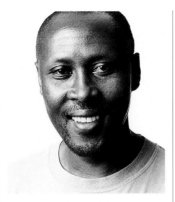

TAYO OLUGBO

osteopath, who has noted a steady improvement. She tends to suffer from asthma, which has eased considerably and she no longer needs daily medication for it.

But, she reports, the greatest gift that tai chi has given her is the ability to cope with the stress and anxiety caused by long hours working at a demanding job. The philosophy of tai chi has enabled her to accept who she is, to feel well grounded, and to move steadily toward her personal and work-related goals. .

Amy Chandler
AGE: 48
Solicitor
BEGAN TAI CHI: Two years ago

Amy encountered tai chi when she was on vacation in Greece at a center for holistic studies. Her 25-year marriage had just ended and she was coming to terms with a second hip replacement. She felt disabled, and this affected her sense of self-worth. She was afraid to face the reality of her new body and she had an aversion to touch. She was feeling numbed by painkilling drugs.

The effects of tai chi were inspiring. Amy immediately sensed that her mind and body were reconnecting and this made her feel as if she had been released from a prison sentence. She continued with tai chi back home. Having found a way to meet her difficulties, she is now far more aware, mentally and physically, feels energized and more alive, and has found strength and happiness.

Tayo Olugbo
AGE: 34
Performer
BEGAN TAI CHI: 15 years ago

Brought up in a rough city district, Tayo had to develop a tough facade in order to survive. He had a fiery temper and he took up kung fu to find a way of channeling it, as well as learning to look after himself. Tayo is big, strong, and fast, but inside, he found all this energy he was generating frightening. At college he tried out tai chi, but soon became bored with the repetitiveness of the exercises.

During his teen years Tayo had learned to love basketball and was playing regularly in a major league. After his move to another town he was accepted to play for the city team, which upgraded him to the national league. But a painful knee was restricting his play. After only three months of tai chi practice he noticed that his knee problem had disappeared. Tayo was persuaded to continue his training. In time, he calmed down enough to be able to discover more about the mental aspects of the art, in particular the quality of stillness.

137

Styles and Schools

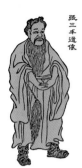

ALTHOUGH THERE IS *only a handful of principal styles of tai chi, each style has many variations, and each variation has many approaches. Deciding what style to learn could therefore be a difficult decision. Pages 8–11 explain the origins of the*

LEFT *The teachers of the past, who evolved different tai chi styles in the 1800s, learned and practiced together.*

different tai chi styles and trace the development of some of their variations and versions. These pages give more information about how these styles and their variations differ, and should give you the information you need when you are trying to choose a style.

CHOOSING A STYLE

In tai chi people who teach or practice may support a particular style or practice wholeheartedly, sometimes even denying the validity of other styles. It is advisable not to heed partisan approaches. Naturally there are arguments for and against each style and each variation, but the similarities between the styles are often more striking, and it is important to realize that the current tendency toward polarization of styles is not how it has always been. The founders of the Yang, Wu, and Hou styles (see pages 10–11) all began by simply studying tai chi. Later, they established a tradition of learning in an atmosphere of collective respect for one another and for their art, which was essentially the application of the yin-yang theory to martial arts. Their intelligence and humility resulted in the collective development of tai chi.

The 20th century saw the spread of tai chi westward. One of the key figures in this dissemination is Cheng Man-ch'ing, who studied Yang style under the grandson of its founder.

Cheng Man-ch'ing altered the Yang Big Form, which had been developed by his teacher, to create a Short Form. After the 1960s this concise version of the Yang form became popular worldwide. Yet Cheng Man-ch'ing did not, perhaps, set out to create a new style. He developed his Short Form as a way of pulling together the essential elements of the art, and in doing this he presented a different way of practicing that was accessible to a wider range of people.

FINDING A CLASS

Tai chi is widespread in Western countries, so it should be possible for most people to find a weekly local class. Remember that it does not matter which style you learn. All are expressions of tai chi. Join the class and learn the style with goodwill. If you later go on to learn a second style, you will find it useful and interesting to have experienced a different approach.

However, if you live in a town or a suburb you may have a bewildering choice. If you are drawn to a certain style, there is no reason why

you should not join a class where it is taught. A more important consideration than style is to find a good environment in which to learn. If you have a choice, try to find a teacher with whom you feel you can make progress, regardless of which school or variation they teach.

If it is difficult to get to a regular class, look for weekend or residential tai chi courses. With the help of this book and perhaps a video you will still be able to practice regularly. Maybe you can find a friend to practice with.

CLASSIC STYLES AND SCHOOLS

Chen style

The first recognized style of tai chi, it is only now becoming popular worldwide. It is characterized by dynamic, physically demanding movements that strengthen the legs and open the hips and other joints. The style clearly demonstrates a polarity of fast and slow, small and large. It is good for anyone wishing to attain a high degree of physical strength and suppleness. It is entirely suitable for beginners.

Yang style

Yang style is perhaps the world's most popular tai chi style. It is often considered the gentlest style, which makes it immediately accessible to the elderly and the not so fit. However, practicing Yang style can result in an extremely fit and agile body. There is more than one version: Big Form (also called Longform) has more postures and takes longer to perform. Beginners usually opt for the Short Form.

Cheng Man-ch'ing style

This popular style, which condenses and softens the longer Yang form, is practiced the world over. This style emphasizes softness and relaxation, making it an especially graceful style, though no less effective as a martial art. It is the style described step by step on pages 62–115.

Wu style

This style, though generally called Wu style, is a small frame version of Yang style, characterized by a forward lean. ("Small frame" means that a shorter stance is adopted than in Yang style, which results in generally smaller body movements.) It is suitable for beginners and for more advanced learners.

Li (Hou) style

This style was devised by Wu Yu-hsiang (see page 11). The style is characterized by a very small frame, with a follow step (this enables you to cover ground with a small stance, so that two or three small steps would be equal to one long stance). It is not as widely taught as Yang and Cheng Man-ch'ing styles.

COMPETITION

For many people, tai chi is a sport, with regular competitive events, in which people can put their solo and partner skills to the test in a potentially stressful situation. Competitions can be valuable forums for interclub or interculturral exchange, when people who practice tai chi have an opportunity to meet and trade views, approaches, and techniques. Some schools are specifically geared to competitive events.

Sun style

Sun Lu-t'ang, a master of Chinese internal martial arts, founded this style, which is characterized by small circular movements and high stances. Because you perform the postures in a normal walking position, you do not use energy getting into a lower stance.

MODERN STYLES AND SCHOOLS

Peking (Beijing) style

This style, devised in the late 1940s by Master Li T'ien-shih, is fairly widely taught. It was conceived as an accessible short form that would raise the health of the Chinese people. The founders also created a standard style that would cater for the rising interest in tai chi as a competitive sport. There is a 24-step form, in which the essential elements of Yang style are condensed. A 36-step form was created, but did not catch on. The 48-step style, which combines the essential elements of Chen, Yang, Wu, and Hou styles, is a standard competition form, and there is an 88-step form.

ASSESSING TEACHERS

The best advice is: stop worrying, but be alert, and do ask questions. When you have located a class, go along early and speak to the teacher. Ask if you can watch the class, or join in. Find out from whom each teacher has learned and how long they have been studying tai chi – considerably more than three years is the ideal.

Ask the teacher to explain what the class offers – not only what style is taught but how it is organized and what happens in it. When you walk into a class, ask yourself whether it resonates well with you.

People sometimes advise looking for a teacher who belongs to a recognized body. This is a good way of finding a teacher. However, it is most important that he or she is alert to your personal needs. Some excellent teachers belong to no recognized body, and there are some teachers on the lists of respected tai chi organizations who may never communicate well with you. You need a teacher who inspires you.

TEACHER TRAINING

Up to now, tai chi has had no gradings or recognizable stages of development. Students would become teachers if and when their own teachers considered it appropriate. Now, however, new standards are evolving and specialist magazines, such as the American publication *Tai Chi*, publish information about new developments. In the UK, a proposal is being considered to introduce a five-year teacher training syllabus, coordinated by the Tai Chi Union of Great Britain.

Further Reading/Useful Addresses

The FOLLOWING SELECTION *of publications is suggested to interested readers in order to offer them the opportunity to expand their understanding of aspects of Tai Chi. Locating a reputable, registered practitioner is best done through a professional association or council.*

TAI CHI

CHEN WEI-MING *Tai Chi Chuan Ta Wen (Questions and Answers on Tai Chi Chuan),* translated by Ben Lo and Robert Smith, North Atlantic Books, 1985.

CHENG MAN-CH'ING *Advanced Tai Chi Form Instructions,* translated by Douglas Wile, Sweet Chi Press, New York, 1989.

CHENG MAN-CH'ING *Cheng Tzu's Thirteen Treatises on Tai Chi Chuan,* translated by Ben Lo and Martin Inn, North Atlantic Books, 1993.

CHENG MAN-CH'ING *T'ai Chi Ch'uan,* North Atlantic Books, 1993.

CROMPTON, PAUL *The Elements of Tai Chi,* Element Books, 1990.

DOCHERTY, DAN *Complete T'ai Chi Ch'uan,* Crowood Press, 1997.

LO, BENJAMIN *The Essence of Tai Chi Chuan: The Literary Tradition,* North Atlantic Books, 1993.

PECK, ALAN *T'ai Chi: The Essential Introductory Guide,* Vermilion, 1999.

SUTTON, NIGEL *Applied T'ai Chi Ch'uan,* A & C Black, 1991.

In Chinese

YANG CHENG-FU *Yang-style T'ai Chi Ch'uan* (recorded by his disciples), Taiping Book Co., Hong Kong, 1976.

ZHANG SAN-FENG *The Secret f Training, the Internal Elixir of the Taiji Art.* Preserved by Taiyi Shanren. Reprinted from ancient text by Anhua Publications, Hong Kong.

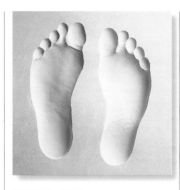

MARTIAL ARTS

FINN, MICHAEL *Martial Arts: A Complete Illustrated History,* Stanley Paul, 1988. Available from Elite Martial Academy, 17A Filmer Road, London SW6 7BU, UK.

WING, R.L. (ED) *The Art of Strategy,* Thorsons, London, and Doubleday & Co, USA, 1998.

QIGUNG

FRANTZIS, BRUCE KUMAR *Opening the Energy Gates of Your Body,* North Atlantic Books, 1997.

CHINESE PHILOSOPHY AND DAOISM

FUNG YU-LAN *A Short History of Chinese Philosophy,* The Free Press, 1995.

LAO TZU *Tao Te Ching,* translated by D.C. Lau, Penguin Books, 1998.

LAO TZU *Tao Te Ching,* translated by Richard Wilhelm, Arkana, 1998.

LAO TZU *Tao Te Ching,* translated by M.H. Kwok et al, Element Books, 1998.

WILHELM, RICHARD (rendered into English by Cary F. Baynes) *I Ching,* Arkana, 1999.

WING, R.L. *The Illustrated I Ching,* Aquarian Press, 1987. This translation is very readable.

HEALING

ANODEA, JUDITH *Wheels of Life, A User's Guide to the Chakra System,* Llewellyn Publications, 1990.

MITCHELL, STEWART *Naturopathy – Understanding the Healing Power of Nature,* Element Books, 1998.

Acknowledgments

Picture credits:
BRIDGEMAN ART LIBRARY: *pp:10,40,140.*
CHARLES WALKER PHOTOGRAPHIC: *p.9B.*
CORBIS: *p.122.*
FORTEAN PICTURE LIBRARY: *p.117T.*
GETTY ONE STONE:
pp:16T,18,19T,22,32,39,44T,118.
IMAGE BANK: *p.120.*
IMAGE STATE: *p.131C.*
HUTCHISON LIBRARY: *p.6T.*

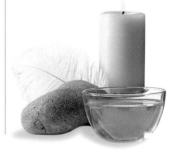

EUROPE

Taijiquan and Qigong Federation for Europe
Web: www.taijiquan-qigung.com

FRANCE

Fédération Française des Tai Chi Chuan Traditionnels
78 Rue Saint Honoré
75001 Paris. Tel: 01 45 43 03 96

THE NETHERLANDS

Pierre de Cat
Postbus 2271800,
AE Alcmaar.
Email: mailing@taijiquan-qigong.com

Stichting Taijiquan Nederland
Postbus 13 26 4, 3507 LG Utrecht.
Tel: 030 289 6336.
Publishers of Nieuwsbrief magazine.

UK

Angus Clark – School of Living Movement
Courses and classes in the UK and worldwide. Tel:+44 [0] 1647 231477
Email: angus@livingmovement.com
Web: www.livingmovement.com

Alan Peck – Natural Way Tai Chi School
c/o Lam Rim Centre,
12 Victoria Place,
Bedminster,
Bristol.

Tai Chi Union for Great Britain
69 Kilpatrick Gardens,
Clarkston, Glasgow G76 7RF.
Tel: +44 [0] 141 810 3482
Email: secretary@taichiunion.com
Publishers of T'ai Chi Ch'uan magazine.

USA

Universal Tai Chi Chuan Association
Contact: Ben Lo
2901 Clement Street,
San Francisco,
CA 94121.

William Chen
2 Washington Square Village
#10J, New York,
N Y10012.
Tel: [212] 675 2816

Yang's Martial Arts Association
Contact: Dr. Yang Jwing Ming
28 Hyde Park Avenue,
Jamaica Plain,
MA 02130-4132.
Tel: [1-617] 524 8892

TAI CHI MAGAZINES

These magazines give useful information about developments and activities in the tai chi world, provide interesting reading, and are the best way to find classes, teachers and other contacts.

Journal of Asian Martial Arts
Media Publishing Co,
821 West 24th Street,
Erie, PA 16502, USA.
Email: info@goviamedia.com
Web: www.goviamedia.com

Qi Magazine: PO Box 116,
Manchester M20 3YN, UK.
Web: www.qimagazine.com

Qi – The Journal of Traditional Eastern Health and Fitness
Insight Graphics Inc,
Box 18476, Anaheim Hills,
CA 92817, USA.
Web: www.qi-journal.com

Nieuwsbrief: published by Stichting Taijiquan Nederland

Tai Chi – The Leading International Magazine of Tai Chi Chuan
Wayfarer Publications, 2601 Siver Ridge Avenue, Los Angeles, CA 90039, USA.
Web: www.tai-chi.com

Tai Chi and Alternative Health
PO Box 6404, London, E18 1EX, UK.
Tel: +44[0] 20 8502 9307

T'ai Chi Ch'uan: published by the Tai Chi Union for Great Britain

Tai Chi International: St Vincent's Publishing, PO Box 460, Thorney, Peterborough, Cambridgeshire PE6 0TQ, UK Tel: [01733] 270 072
Email: tcinter@easynet.co.uk

Tai Chi Magazine: published by the Fédération Française des Tai Chi Chuan Traditionnels

HOLISTIC VACATIONS / RETREATS

These three centers offer tai chi in their programs. All are located in Europe but have an international reputation.

Skyros, Greece
Tel: +44 [0] 207 267 4424
Email: Skyros@easynet.co.uk
Web: www.skyros.com

La Serrania, Mallorca, Spain
Tel: +34 639 306 432
Fax: +34 971 182 144
Web: www.laserrania.com

Cortijo Romero, Spain
Email: bookings@cortijo-romero.co.uk
Web: www.cortijo-romero.co.uk

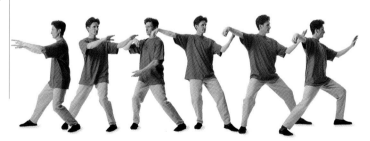

Index